D0478731

# Atlas of
# MIGRAINE
## AND OTHER HEADACHES
### Second Edition

# Atlas of
# MIGRAINE
# AND OTHER HEADACHES
## Second Edition

Edited by

Stephen D Silberstein MD
M Alan Stiles DMD
William B Young MD

Jefferson Headache Center
Thomas Jefferson University
Philadelphia, Pennsylvania, USA

informa
healthcare

New York London

First published in the United Kingdom under the title An Atlas of Headache in 2002 by Parthenon Publishing
This edition published by Taylor & Francis,
an imprint of the Taylor & Francis Group,
2 Park Square, Milton Park
Abingdon, Oxon OX14 4RN

Tel.: +44 (0)20 7017 6000
Fax.: +44 (0)20 7017 6699
Website: www.tandf.co.uk



British Library Cataloguing in Publication Data

Data available on application

Library of Congress Cataloging-in-Publication Data

Data available on application

ISBN 1-84214-273-9

Distributed in North and South America by

Taylor & Francis
2000 NW Corporate Blvd
Boca Raton, FL 33431, USA

*Within Continental USA*
Tel: 800 272 7737; Fax: 800 374 3401
*Outside Continental USA*
Tel: 561 994 0555; Fax: 561 361 6018
E-mail: orders@crcpress.com

Distributed in the rest of the world by
Thomson Publishing Services
Cheriton House
North Way
Andover, Hampshire SP10 5BE, UK
Tel.: +44 (0)1264 332424
E-mail: salesorder.tandf@thomsonpublishingservices.co.uk

Composition by Parthenon Publishing

# Contents

# List of contributors

**Elizabeth W Loder** MD
Spaulding Rehabilitation Hospital
Boston, MA 02114
USA

**Laszlo L Mechtler** MD
Dent Neurologic Institute
200 Sterling Drive
Orchard Park, NY 14127
USA

**Michael L Oshinsky** PhD
Jefferson Headache Center
111 S. 11th Street
Suite 8130 Gibbon Bldg
Philadelphia, PA 19107
USA

**Mario F P Peres** MD
São Paulo Headache Center
R. Maestro Cardim, 887
01323–001
São Paulo 01323-001
Brazil

**Todd D Rozen** MD
Michigan Head-Pain Neurological Institute
3120 Professional Drive
Ann Arbor, MI 48104
USA

**Stephen D Silberstein** MD
Jefferson Headache Center
111 S. 11th Street
Suite 8130 Gibbon Bldg
Philadelphia, PA 19107
USA

**M Alan Stiles** DMD
Jefferson Headache Center
111 S. 11th Street
Suite 8130 Gibbon Bldg
Philadelphia, PA 19107
USA

**William B Young** MD
Jefferson Headache Center
111 S. 11th Street
Suite 8130 Gibbon Bldg
Philadelphia, PA 19107
USA

# Acknowledgements

**Nitamar Abdala**
Federal University of São Paulo
Rua Napoleão de Barros, 800
Vila Clementino
São Paulo, SP, CEP 04024–002
Brazil

**David J Capobianco** MD
Mayo Clinic, Jacksonville
4500 San Pablo Road
Jacksonville, FL 32224
USA

**Gary Carpenter** MD
Jefferson Medical College
1025 Walnut Street
Philadelphia, PA 19107
USA

**Henrique Carrete Jr** MD
Department of Radiology
Universidade Federal de São Paulo
São Paulo
Brazil

**John Edmeads** MD
Sunnybrook Medical Center
University of Toronto
2075 Bayview Avenue
Toronto, Ontario M4N 3M5
Canada

**Deborah I Freidman**
University of Rochester Eye Institute
601 Elmwood Avenue
Rochester, NY 14642
USA

**Peter J Goadsby** MD
Institute of Neurology
National Hospital for Neurology & Neurosurgery
Queen Square
London WC1N 3BG
UK

**Richard Hargreaves** PhD
Pharmacology and Imaging
Merck Research Laboratories
Merck & Co, Inc
WP 42–300
770 Sumneytown Pike
P.O. Box 4
West Point, PA 19486
USA

**Bernadette Jaeger** DDS
Section of Oral Medicine and Orofacial Pain
School of Dentistry
University of California, Los Angeles
Los Angeles, CA 90064–1782
USA

**Marco A Lana-Peixoto** MD
Federal University of Minas Gerais
Medical School
Rua Padre Rolim 769 – 13° andar
Belo Horizonte - MG 30130–090
Brazil

**Richard B Lipton** MD
Department of Neurology
Albert Einstein College of Medicine
1165 Morris Park Avenue
Rousso Building, Room 332
Bronx, NY 10461
USA

**Suzana M F Malheiros** MD
Department of Neurology
Universidade Federal de São Paulo
São Paulo
Brazil

**Pericles de Andrade Maranhão-Filho** MD MSc PhD
Federal University of Rio de Janeiro
Clementino Fraga Filho Hospital
National Institute of Cancer
Rio de Janeiro
Brazil

**Andrew A Parsons** PhD
Head Migraine & Stroke Research
GlaxoSmithKline
Neurology Centre of Excellence
for Drug Discovery
New Frontiers Science Park
Harlow, Essex
UK

**Julio Pascual** MD
University Hospital 'Marqués de Valdecilla'
Avda. Valdecilla
39008 Santander
Spain

**Luiz Paulo de Queiroz** MD MSc
Clinica do Cerebro
Rua Presidente Coutinho, 464
88015–231 Florianopolis, SC
Brazil

**Margarita Sanchez del Rio** MD
Neurology Department
Fundación Hospital Alcorcón
Juan Carlos I University
Alcorcón, Madrid
Spain

**Germany Goncalves Veloso** MD
Department of Neurology
Federal University of São Paulo
São Paulo
Brazil

**Paul Winner** DO FAAN
Palm Beach Headache Center
Nova Southeastern University
5205 Greenwood Avenue
West Palm Beach, FL 33407
USA

**Vera Lucia Faria Xavier** MD
Headache Center
Santo Amaro University
São Paulo
Brazil

The image on the front cover is of the sculpture "Headache Man" by Wesley Andregg and is displayed at the Sniderman Gallery, Philadelphia. Reproduced with permission.

# Preface

It is rare for medical students to have more than one lecture on headache management during their education, and residents in training, even in neurology, rarely get any more formal training. We have tried, through this Atlas, to demonstrate the problem of headache from a visual perspective. For many, learning from pictures and diagrams is educational and more enjoyable than through the printed word. By presenting information on headache in a visual format, we hope to educate caregivers to better recognize head pain complaints and ultimately provide better care for patients.

Chronic head and face pain may be either a result of numerous disorders or a symptom of a more ominous secondary cause. Correct diagnosis is essential for proper treatment.

To assist the clinician, we include the history of headache, its epidemiology, diagnosis, and treatment. We address migraine, tension-type, and cluster headache, in addition to the rare or more unusual primary and secondary headache disorders. We have tried to include classic images from other texts, as well as new images that illustrate the disorders and reflect the most current thinking. This compilation of slides, images, graphs, paintings, and drawings has been obtained from physicians from all over the world.

We would like to thank the many physicians and researchers who have contributed to the success of this Atlas. Without their willingness to share their images and data we would not be able to present this topic in this format. We hope that this edition of the Atlas offers an overview of the numerous disorders that cause head pain, provides a better understanding for those treating these disorders, and results in better care for those who suffer with these disorders.

*Stephen D Silberstein*
*M Alan Stiles*
*William B Young*

# Foreword

In medieval maps, the periphery of the world was shrouded in mystery with vivid images of hypothetical dragons lurking at the edges. One might suspect that an atlas about migraine and other headaches would be rife with such dragons, as not all of the headache world has been completely charted. How does one see a headache? How does one map a headache?

The present authors are to be commended for presenting an 'Illustrated Migraine and other Headaches News' for our information and enjoyment. The common headache entities of migraine, cluster and tension-type headaches as well as the more sinister structural causes of headache are outlined in the text to provide a framework on which to hang the illustrations – some scientific, some historical and some artistic. This display makes for a relaxed approach to a complex subject like ambling through an art gallery to view an exhibition that conveys a message. It is a pathway well worth taking for pleasure as well as enlightenment.

*James W Lance*
*Emeritus Professor of Neurology*
*University of New South Wales*
*Sydney, Australia*
*Past President of the*
*International Headache Society*

# 1

# Historical aspects of headache

Stephen D Silberstein

## HEADACHE IN THE ANCIENT WORLD

Headache has troubled mankind from the dawn of civilization. Signs of trepanation, a procedure wherein the skull was perforated with an instrument, are evident on neolithic human skulls dating from 7000–3000 BC[1] (Figures 1.1 and 1.2). Originally, it was thought that the procedure had been performed to release demons and evil spirits, but recent evidence suggests that it was carried out for medical reasons[2]. Trepanation continues to be practiced today, without anesthesia, by some African tribes. It is primarily performed for relief of headache or removal of a fracture line after head injury[3].

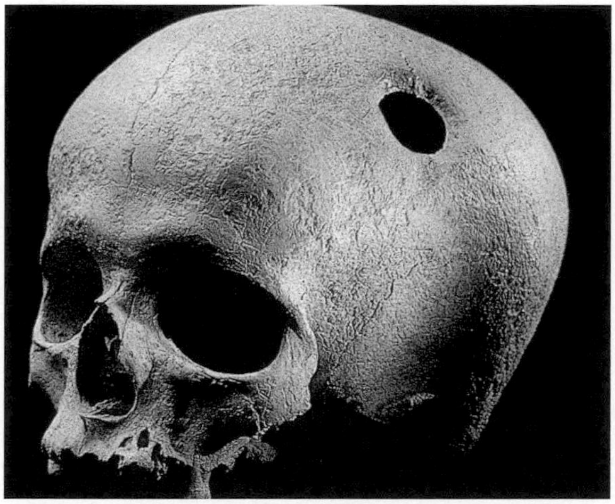

**Figure 1.1** Trepanned skull, approximately 3000 years old. Of course, we do not know why this individual had trepanation. He did, however, survive long enough (this is 1000 BC) to generate new bone growth at the margin of the trepanned hole. Reproduced with kind permission of John Edmeads

Headache prescriptions written on papyrus (Figure 1.3) were already known in ancient Egypt. The Ebers Papyrus, dated circa 1200 BC and said to be based on medical documents from 2500 BC, describes migraine, neuralgia and shooting head pains[4]. It was

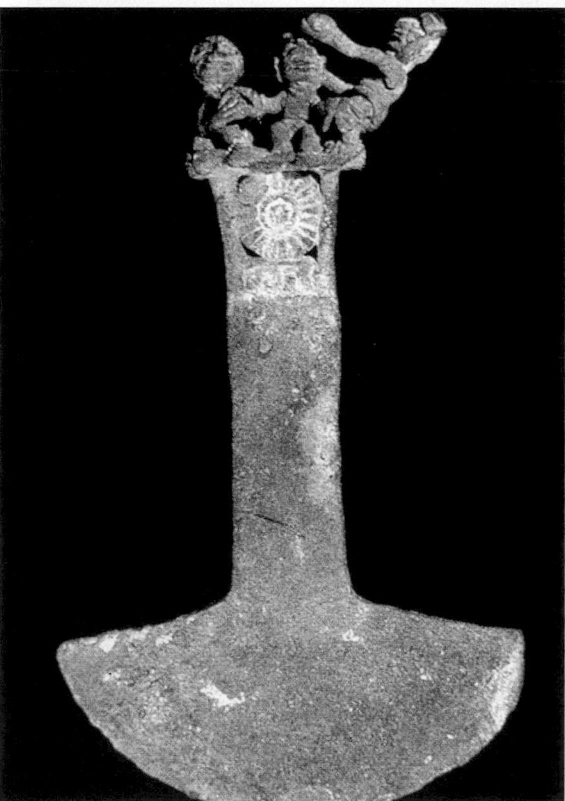

**Figure 1.2** Trepanation has been performed around the world. This is a tumi, a pre-Columbian trepan from Peru. Note the instructions for use on top of the handle. Reproduced with kind permission of John Edmeads

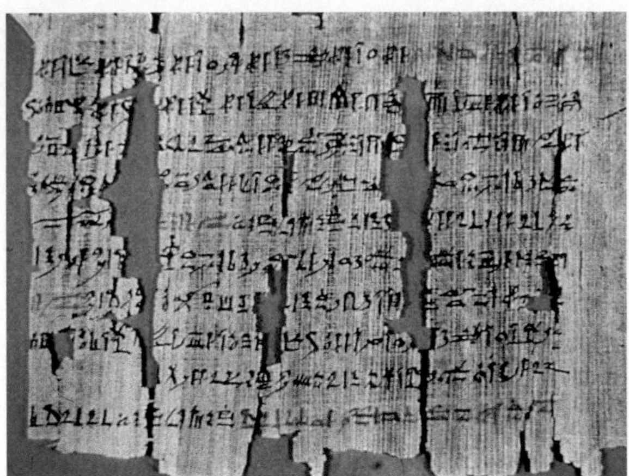

**Figure 1.3** Papyrus from Thebes, Egypt (2500 BC). Now in a British museum. It is totally illegible, and therefore instantly recognizable as a prescription

practice at the time to firmly bind a clay crocodile holding grain in its mouth to the patient's head using a strip of linen that bore the names of the gods[5,6] (Figure 1.4). This technique may have produced headache relief by compressing and cooling the scalp[5].

Hippocrates (470–410 BC, Figure 1.5) described a shining light, usually in the right eye, followed by violent pain that began in the temples and eventually reached the entire head and neck area[5]. He believed that headache could be triggered by exercise or intercourse[6], that migraine resulted from vapors rising from the stomach to the head and that vomiting could partially relieve the pain of headache[5,6]. Celsus (AD 215–300) believed 'drinking wine, or crudity [dyspepsia] or cold, or heat of a fire or the sun' could trigger migraine. Because of his classic descriptions, Aretaeus of Cappodocia (second century AD) is credited with discovering migraine headache. The term 'migraine' itself is derived from the Greek word 'hemicrania', introduced by Galen in approximately AD 200. He mistakenly believed it was caused by the ascent of vapors, either excessive, too hot or too cold. Clearly, migraine was well known in the ancient world[4].

## HEADACHE OVER THE CENTURIES

In the twelfth century, Abbess Hildegard of Bingen described her visions (Figure 1.6), later attributed to her migraine aura, in terms that are both mystical and apocalyptic[7]:

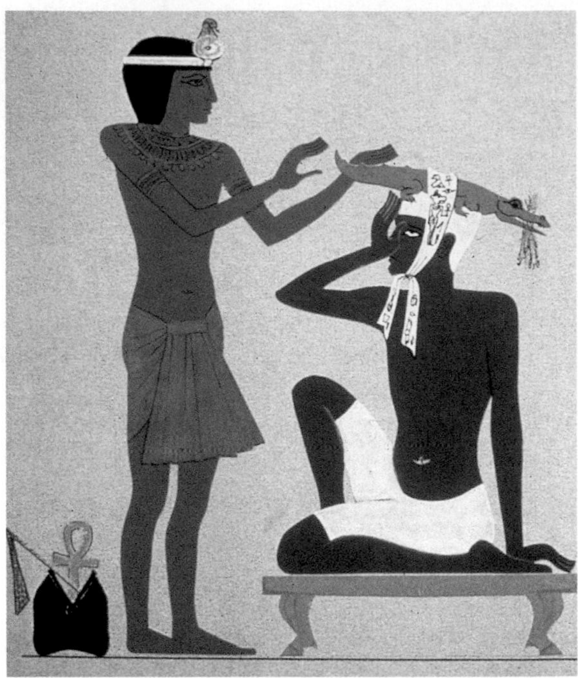

**Figure 1.4** Cartoon, translating above papyrus: 'The physician shall take a crocodile made of clay, with sacred grain in its mouth, and an eye of faience. He shall bind it to the head of the patient with a strip of fine linen upon which is written the names of the Gods. And the physician shall pray'

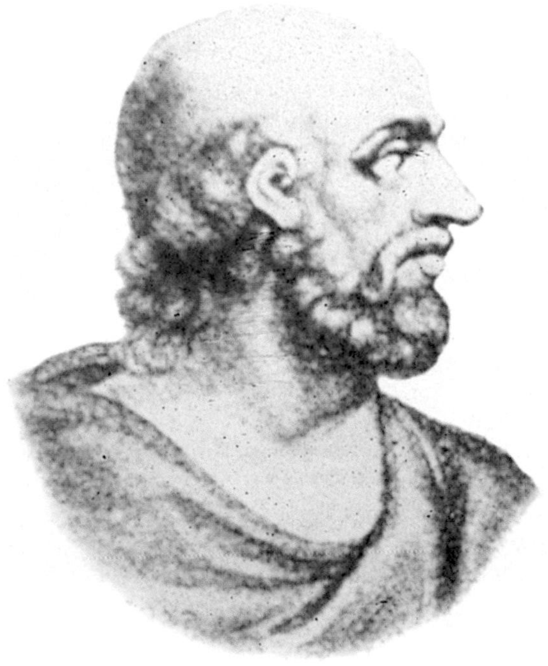

**Figure 1.5** Hippocrates described migraine circa 400 BC. Courtesy of the National Library of Medicine, Bethesda, USA

*'I saw a great star, most splendid and beautiful, and with it an exceeding multitude of falling sparks with which the star followed southward ... and suddenly they were all annihilated, being turned into black coals ... and cast into the abyss so that I could see them no more'.*

In 1667 Thomas Willis (Figures 1.7 and 1.8) brilliantly described a woman with severe, periodic, migrainous headache preceded by a prodrome and associated with vomiting[4]:

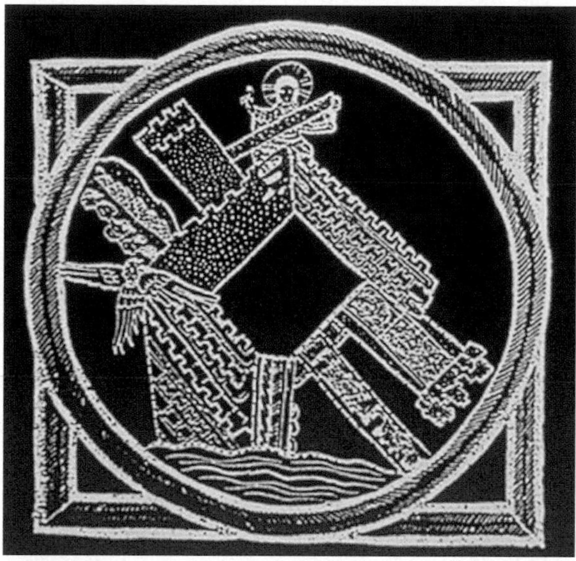

**Figure 1.6** 'Vision of the Heavenly City' from a manuscript of Hildegard's Scivias written at Bingen (circa AD 1180)

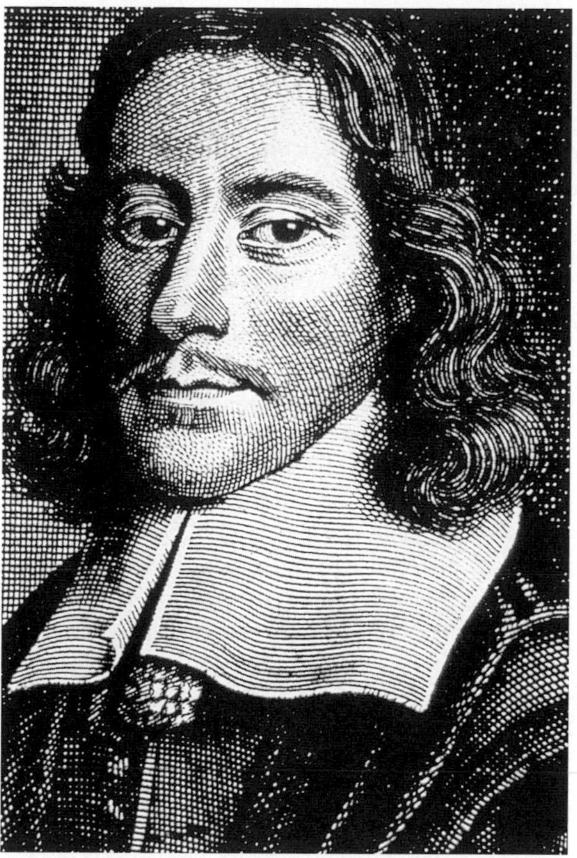

**Figure 1.7** Thomas Willis (1621–75), the father of neurology. The first to postulate that 'megrim' was due to blood 'estuating' (stagnating) in the dural vessels, distending them and producing head pain. Courtesy of the National Library of Medicine, Bethesda, USA

3. As to the differences of the Headach, the common diſtinction is, That the pain of the Head is either without the Skull, or within its cavity: The former is a more rare and a more gentle diſeaſe, becauſe the parts above the Skull are not ſo ſenſible as the interior *Meninges*; nor are they watered with ſo plentiful a flood of Blood, that by its ſudden and vehement incurſion, they may be eaſily diſtended, or inflamed above meaſure. Secondly, The other kind of Headach, to wit, within the Skull, is more frequent, and much more cruel, becauſe the Membranes, cloathing the Brain, are very ſenſible, and the Blood is poured upon them by a manifold paſſage, and by many and greater Arteries. Further, becauſe the Blood or its Serum, ſometimes paſſing thorow all the Arteries at once, both the *Carotides* and the *Vertebrals*, and ſometimes apart, thorow theſe or thoſe, on the one ſide or the oppoſite, bring hurt to the *Meninges*, hence the pain is cauſed that is interior; which is either univerſal, infeſting the whole Head or its greateſt part; or particular, which is limited to ſome private region; and ſometimes produces a Meagrim on the ſide, ſometimes in the forepart; and ſometimes in the hinder part of the Head.

**Figure 1.8** Original publication of Thomas Willis' work, *The London Practice of Physick*. He stated that migraine was caused by vasodilation

*'... beautiful and young woman, imbued with a slender habit of body, and an hot blood, was wont to be afflicted with frequent and wandering fits of headache ... On the day before the coming of the spontaneous fit of this disease, growing very hungry in the evening, she ate a most plentiful supper, with an hungry, I may say a greedy appetite; presaging by this sign, that the pain of the head would most certainly follow the next morning; and the event never failed this augury ... she was troubled also with vomiting'.*

Migraine was distinguished from common headache by Tissot in 1783[8], who ascribed it to a supraorbital neuralgia '... provoked by reflexes from the stomach, gallbladder or uterus'. Over the next century, DuBois Reymond, Mollendorf and, later, Eulenburg proposed different vascular theories for migraine. In the late eighteenth century, Erasmus Darwin (Figure 1.9), grandfather of Charles Darwin, suggested treating headache by centrifugation. He believed headaches were caused by vasodilation, and suggested placing the patient in a centrifuge to force the blood from the head to the feet[5,6]. Fothergill in 1778 introduced the term 'fortification spectra' to describe the typical visual aura or disturbance of migraine. Fothergill used the term 'fortification'[6] because the visual aura resembled a fortified town surrounded with bastions[9,10].

In 1873, Liveing (Figure 1.10) wrote the first monograph on migraine, entitled *On Megrim, Sick-headache, and Some Allied Disorders: A Contribution to the Pathology of Nerve-storms*, and originated the neural theory of migraine. He ascribed the problem to '... disturbances of the autonomic nervous system', which he called 'nerve storms'[9]. William Gowers, in 1888, published an influential neurology textbook, *A Manual of Disease of the Nervous System*[10]. Gowers emphasized the importance of a healthy lifestyle and advocated using a solution of nitroglycerin (1% in alcohol), combined with other agents, to treat headaches. The remedy later became known as the 'Gowers mixture'. Gowers was also famous for recommending Indian hemp (marijuana) for headache relief[5,6].

Lewis Carroll described migrainous phenomena in *Alice in Wonderland* and *Through the Looking Glass*, depicting instances of central scotoma,

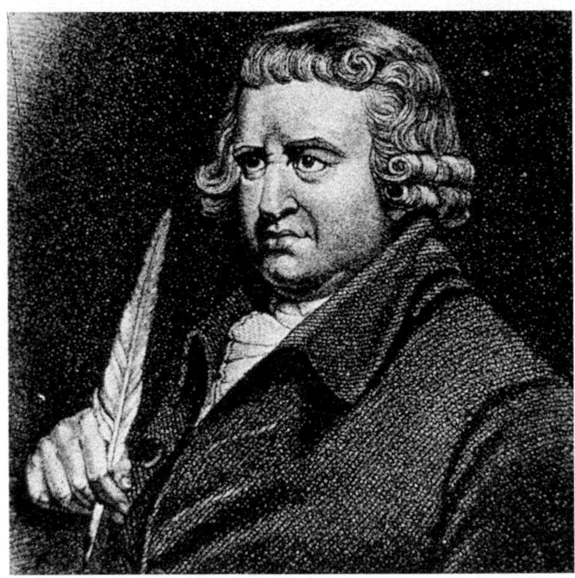

**Figure 1.9** Erasmus Darwin (1731–1802), Charles' grandfather, a physician, lived in the eighteenth century. He postulated that since migraine, as Willis suggested, was due to too much blood in the head, ideal treatment would be to construct a giant centrifuge, put the patient in it and spin him. As the blood left the head, the headache should disappear. Fortunately, the technology was not available to mount the experiment. Courtesy of the National Library of Medicine, Bethesda, USA

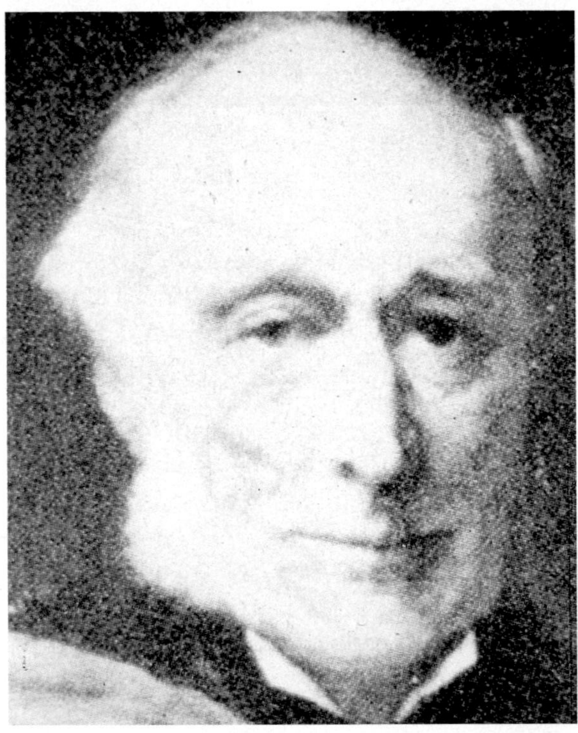

**Figure 1.10** Edward Liveing (1832–1919), the author of an influential book on migraine in 1873, who argued that 'megrim' was a 'nerve-storm' or epileptic manifestation

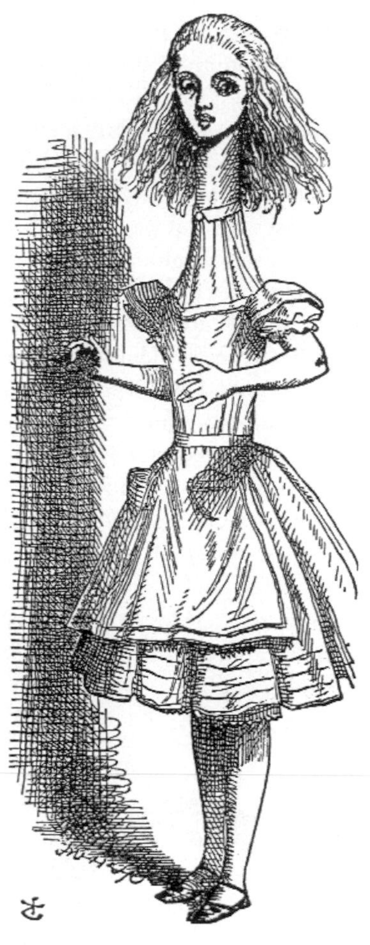

**Figure 1.11** Illustration by John Tenniel from Alice in Wonderland. Was Lewis Carroll writing his migraine auras into his book?

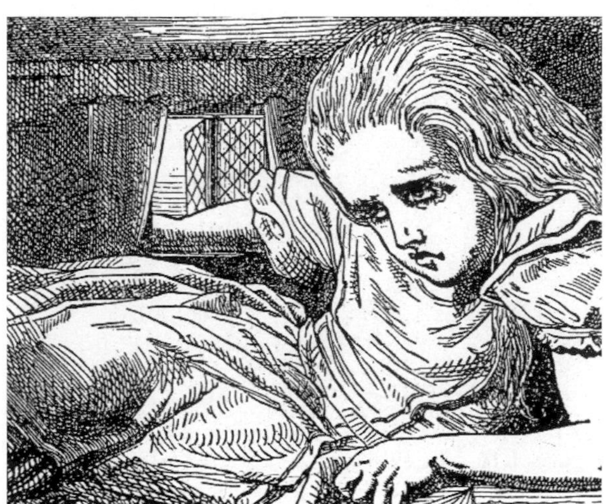

**Figure 1.12** Illustration by John Tenniel from Alice in Wonderland. The image depicts the sense of being too large for one's surroundings

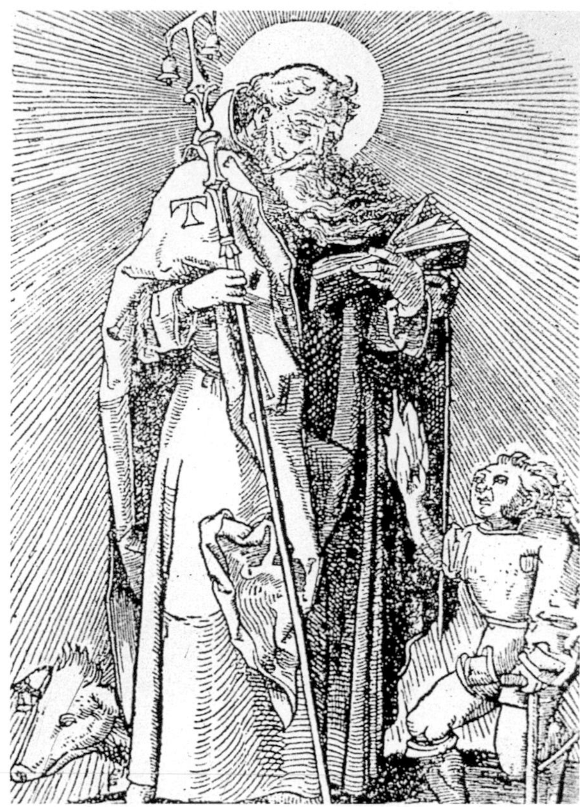

**Figure 1.13** Saint Anthony. Note the patient who has lost limbs as a result of gangrene due to ergotism (eating bread made from rye contaminated with ergot fungus). Limbs turned black, as though charred by fire, then fell off. Hence the term 'St. Anthony's Fire'. If you prayed to Saint Anthony, your symptoms might improve. Note Anthony's pet pig. Courtesy of the National Library of Medicine, Bethesda, USA

tunnel vision, phonophobia, vertigo, distortions in body image, dementia and visual hallucinations (Figures 1.11 and 1.12).

Greek and Roman ancient writings include references to 'blighted grains' and 'blackened bread', and to the use of concoctions of powdered barley flower to hasten childbirth. During the Middle Ages, written accounts of ergot poisoning first appeared. Epidemics were described in which the characteristic symptom was gangrene of the feet, legs, hands and arms, often associated with burning sensations in the extremities. The disease was known as 'Ignis Sacer' or 'Holy Fire' and, later, as 'St. Anthony's Fire', in honor of the saint at whose shrine relief was obtained. This relief probably resulted from the use of a diet free of contaminated grain during the pilgrimage to the shrine (Figure 1.13)[11]. The term 'ergot' is derived from the French word 'argot'

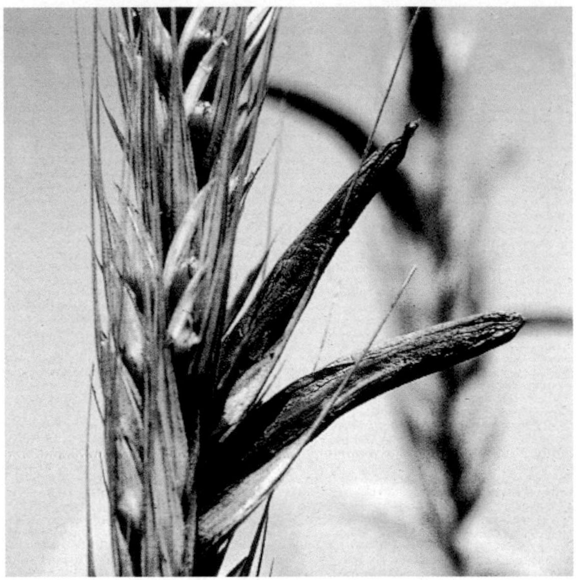

**Figure 1.14** A stalk of grain upon which are growing two purple excrescences – *Claviceps purpurea*, or 'ergot fungus'. Reproduced with kind permission of John Edmeads

meaning 'rooster's spur'. It describes the small, banana-shaped sclerotium of the fungus. Louis René Tulasne of Paris in 1853 established that ergot was not a hypertrophied rye seed, but a fungus having three stages in one life cycle, and he named it *Claviceps purpurea* (Figure 1.14). Once infected by the fungus, the rye seed was transformed into a spur-shaped mass of fungal pseudotissue, purple-brown in colour: the resting stage of the fungus, known as the 'sclerotium' (derived from the Greek 'skleros' meaning 'hard')[11]. In 1831, Heinrich Wiggers (Figure 1.15), a pharmacist of Göttingen, Germany tested ergot extracts in animals. Among his models was the 'rooster comb test': a rooster, when fed ergotin, became ataxic and nauseous, acquired a blanched comb and suffered from severe convulsions, dying days later. The 'rooster comb test' continued to be used into the following century by investigators studying the physiologic properties of ergot[11]. Later Woakes, in 1868, reported the use of ergot of rye in the treatment of neuralgia[12]. The earliest reports in

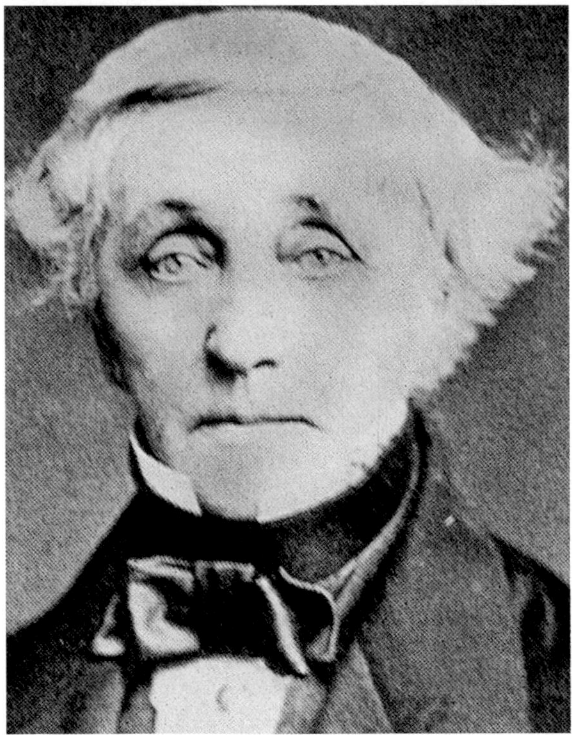

**Figure 1.15** As the botanists argued over the nature of ergot, the chemists were attempting to unravel the mystery of its composition. Heinrich Wiggers (1803–1880), a pharmacist of Göttingen, Germany was probably the first to analyze ergot with the set purpose of trying to isolate the active principle or principles. In 1831 he tested his ergot extracts in animals

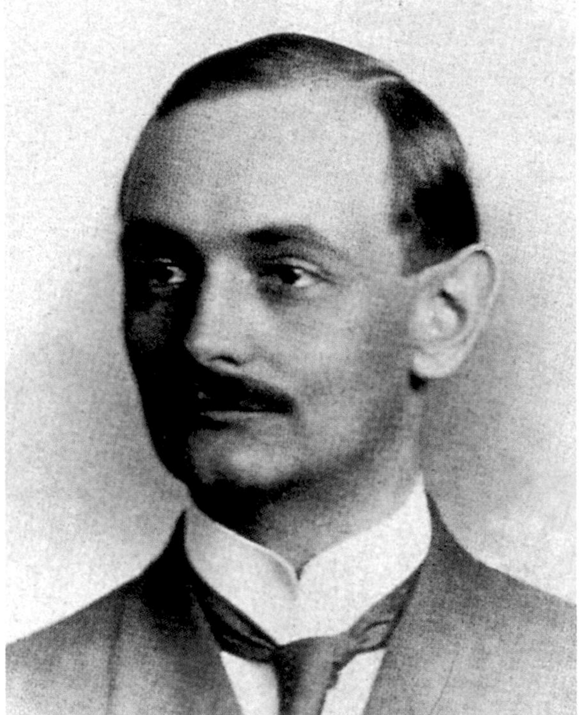

**Figure 1.16** In 1918, Arthur Stoll (1887–1971), a young chemist working in Basel, Switzerland announced the isolation of the first pure crystalline substance, ergotamine. Professor Stoll made many additional contributions to our understanding of ergot, and in 1917 became the founder of the Sandoz 'Department of Pharmaceutical Specialities'

the medical literature on the use of ergot in the treatment of migraine were those of Eulenberg in Germany in 1883, Thomson in the United States in 1894 and Campbell in England in 1894. Stevens' *Modern Materia Medica* mentioned the use of ergot for the treatment of migraine in 1907[13].

The first pure ergot alkaloid, ergotamine, was isolated by Stoll (Figure 1.16) in 1918 and used primarily in obstetrics and gynecology until 1925, when Rothlin successfully treated a case of severe and intractable migraine with a subcutaneous injection of ergotamine tartrate. This indication was pursued vigorously by various researchers over the following decades and was reinforced by the belief in a vascular origin of migraine and the concept that ergotamine tartrate acted as a vasoconstrictor. In 1938, John Graham and Harold Wolff[14] demonstrated that ergotamine worked by constricting blood vessels and used this as proof of the vascular theory of migraine (Figures 1.17 and 1.18).

For further milestones in the history of headache, see Figures 1.19–1.30.

## MODERN HEADACHE TREATMENTS

The modern approach to treating migraine began with the development of sumatriptan by Pat Humphrey and his colleagues[15]. Based on the concept that serotonin can relieve headache, they designed a chemical entity that was similar to serotonin, although more stable and with fewer side-effects. This development led to the modern clinical

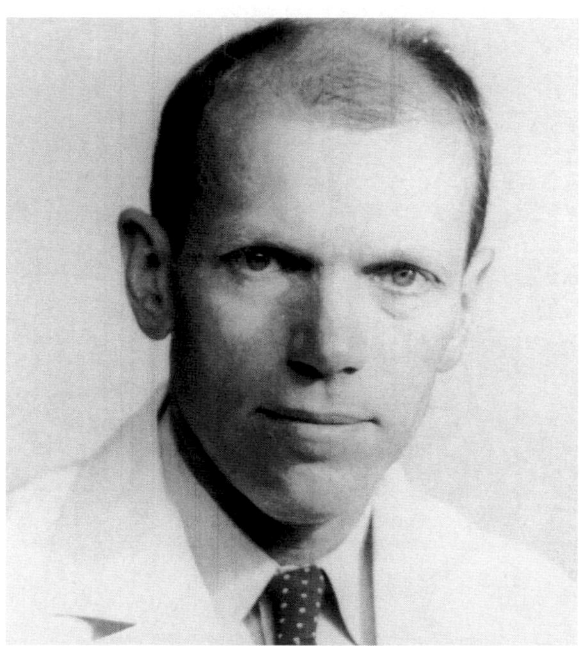

**Figure 1.17** Harold Wolff (1898–1962). He did have the technology to run Darwin's experiment. He borrowed the G-machine at the US Army Air Corps laboratory in 1940. The headache did indeed disappear – as the patient lost consciousness. He is better known for his experiments with ergotamine tartrate (see Figure 1.18). Courtesy of the National Library of Medicine, Bethesda, USA

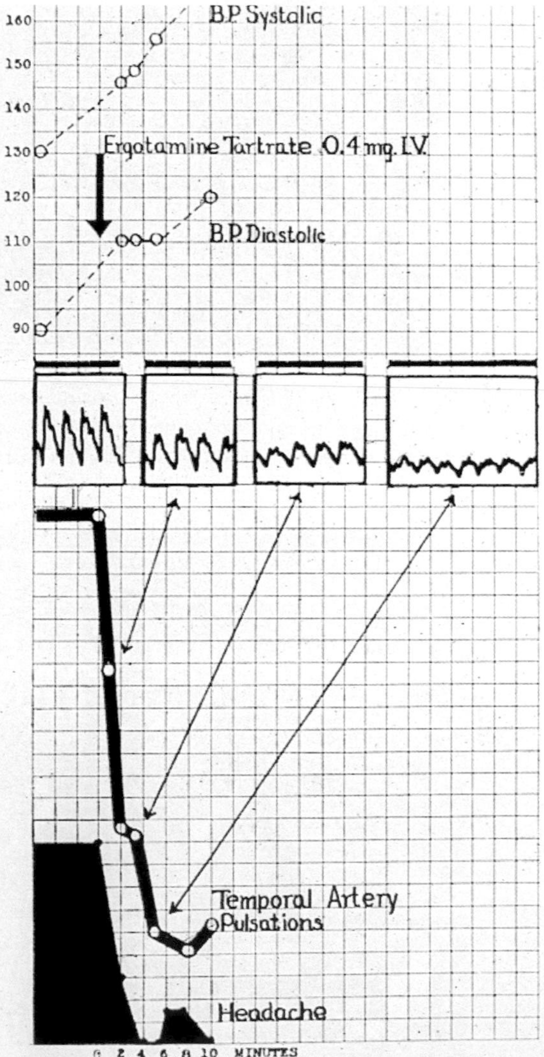


**Figure 1.18** Illustration from Wolff's classic paper on the effect of ergotamine tartrate on pulsatility of cranial blood vessels and on migraine headache. Reproduced with permission from Graham JR, Wolff HG. Mechanisms of migraine headache and action of ergotamine tartrate. *Arch Neurol Psychiatr* 1938; 39:737–63

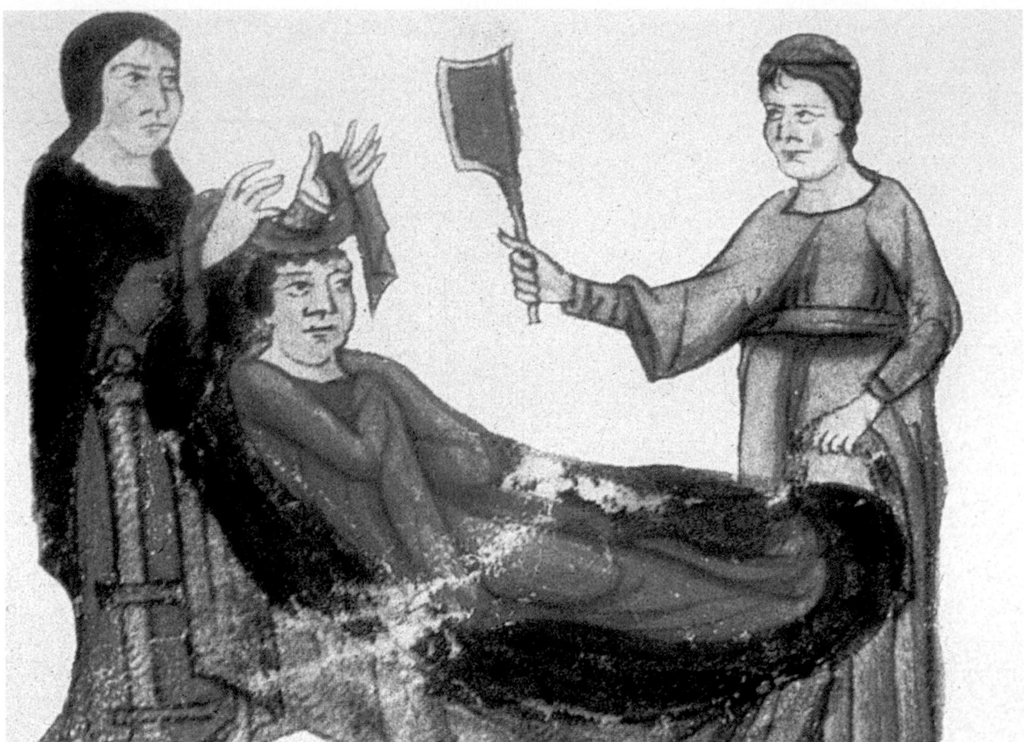

**Figure 1.19** Mural from wall of Roman villa, circa AD 300. The master of the house has migraine. One handmaiden is applying a poultice of honey and opium (did they know back then that there are opioid receptors on peripheral nerves?), and another is fanning the master's brow

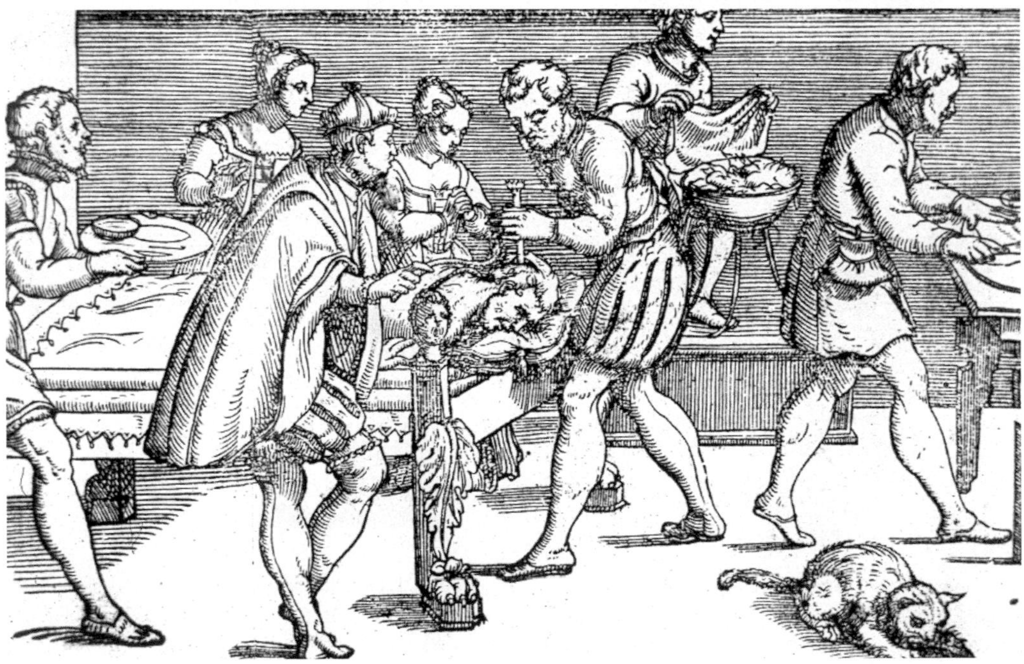

**Figure 1.20** Illustration from Italian medieval manuscript, by Della Croce, dated 1583. The legend indicates that this man was trepanned for hemicrania. Outcome unknown. Note the cat in the lower right hand corner, that has caught a rat (the beginning of the aseptic method in the operating room?)

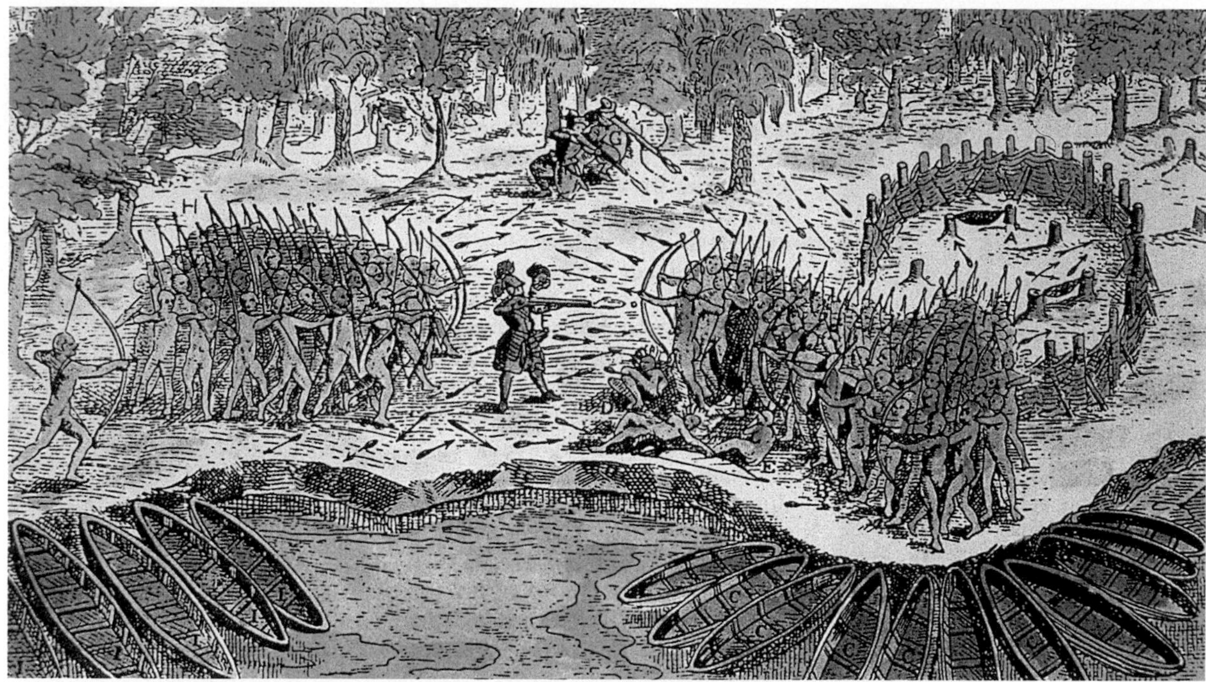

**Figure 1.21** On July 30, 1609, Samuel de Champlain, a French explorer of New France (North America), was taken along by his Huron Indian hosts on a raid against the Mohawks, who lived on the shores of a large lake (Lake Champlain) in what is now upper New York State. There is a drawing by Champlain himself of the battle, in which he and his fellow Frenchmen won the day with their muskets. Towards the end of the battle, Champlain developed a severe migraine. See Figure 1.22

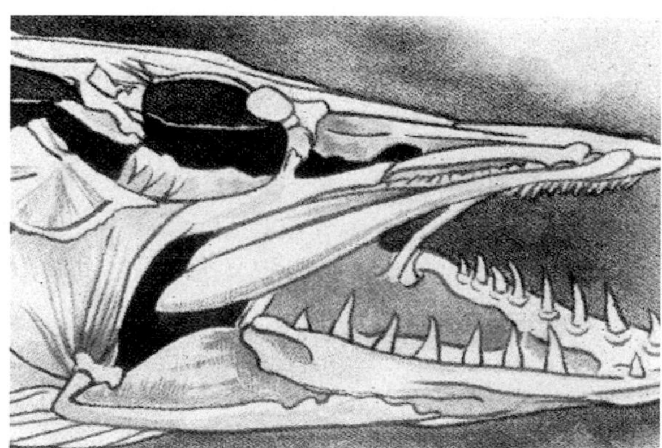

**Figure 1.22** The victorious Hurons caught a gar pike in the lake, stripped its head of the flesh and instructed Champlain to rake his painful head with the sharp teeth, sufficient to draw blood. He did so, and his headache disappeared. Champlain took the head back to France with him, and gave it to the King of France, who also had migraine. We do not know if he ever used it

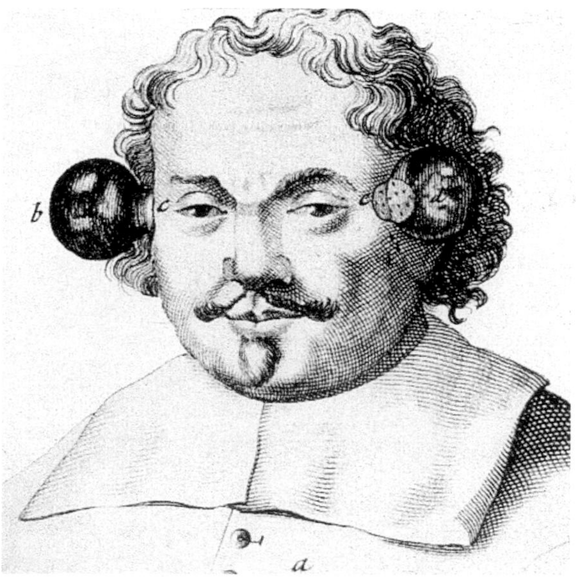


**Figure 1.23** Dutch engraving, seventeenth century. The migraine sufferer has had puncture wounds put into his sore temples. Then heated glass globes are placed with their open mouths over the puncture wounds. As the globes cooled, a vacuum was set up, sucking the blood from the temples into the globes and relieving the headache. In this way, several patients could be treated at once (the first migraine clinic?)

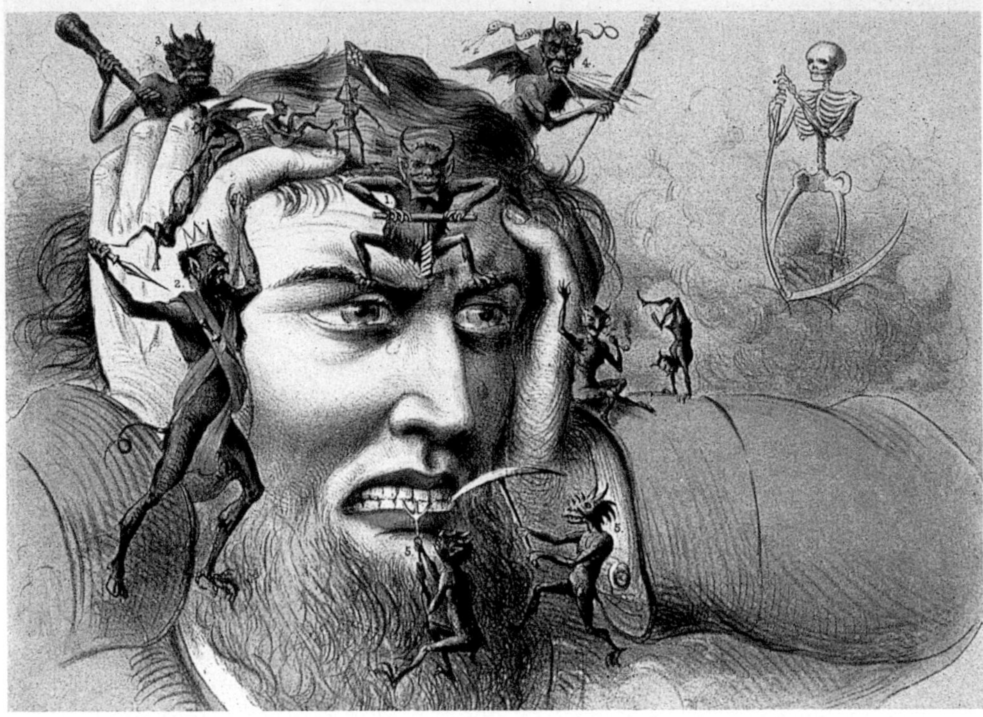


**Figure 1.24** Advertisement from USA popular magazine (Harper's), 1863. Wolcott's Instant Pain Annihilator. Headache before Wolcott's treatment

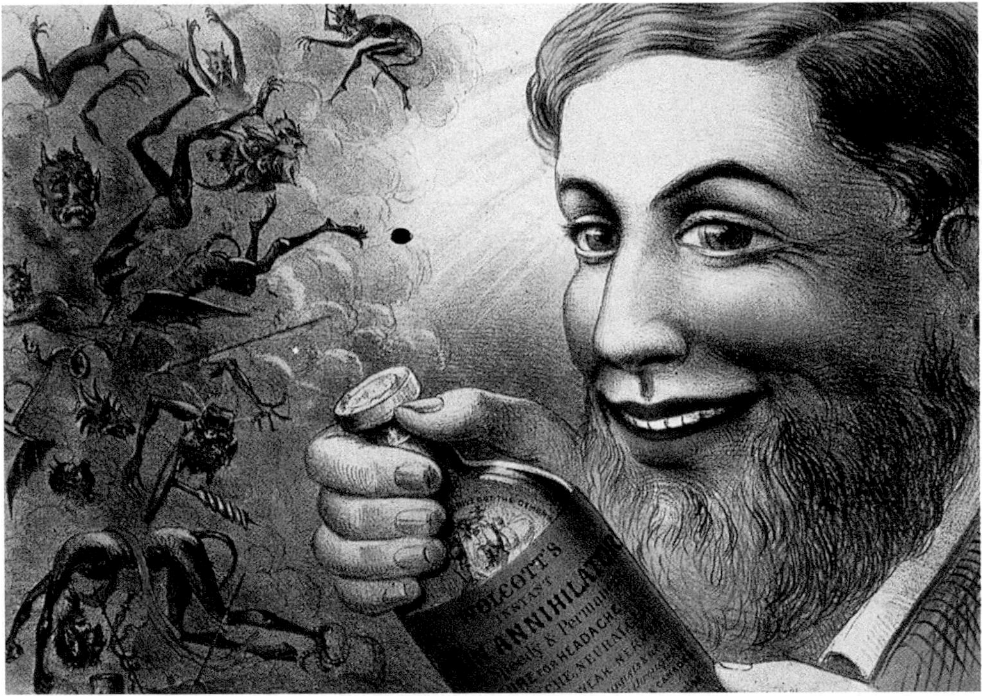

**Figure 1.25** Advertisement continued. Headache gone (possible 2 hour pain relief?) after Wolcott's treatment

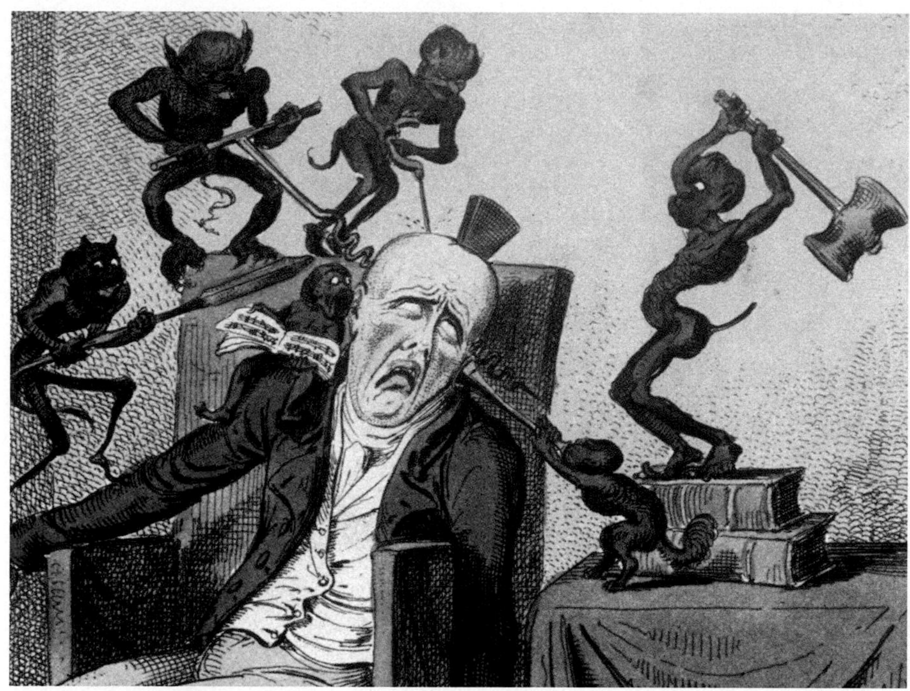

**Figure 1.26** 'Headache'. The colored etching by George Cruikshank (1792–1878) after a design by Maryatt (London, 1819) dramatizes the impact of a headache of such intensity that one might almost venture to diagnose it as migraine. Reproduced with kind permission of Corbis Images, London, UK

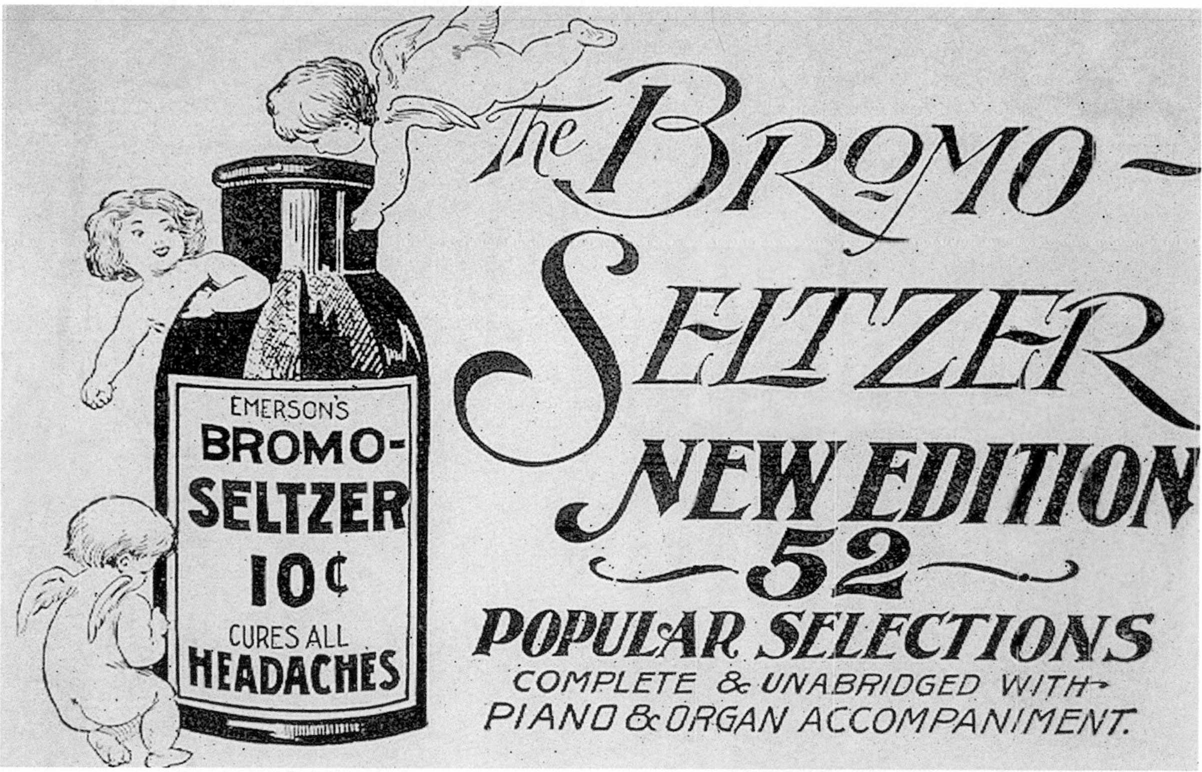


**Figure 1.27** In 1888, Isaac E. Emerson (1859–1937), with his background in chemistry and pharmacy, conceived the idea of a headache remedy in his drugstore in Baltimore. The remedy was a granular effervescent salt he named 'Bromo-Seltzer'. Dispensing it to friends and customers at his drugstore, it soon became so successful that he abandoned his retail business to devote his time to the manufacture of his product. Eventually he established the Emerson Drug Company, incorporating it in Maryland in 1891

trials for acute migraine treatment and to the elucidation of the mechanism of action of what are now called the triptans.

We are at the threshold of an explosion in the understanding, diagnosis and treatment of migraine and other headaches. Many new triptans have been developed and many more will soon be, or are already, available, including zolmitriptan, naratriptan, eletriptan, frovatriptan, rizatriptan and almotriptan. Modern preventive treatment began with the belief that migraine was due to excess sero-

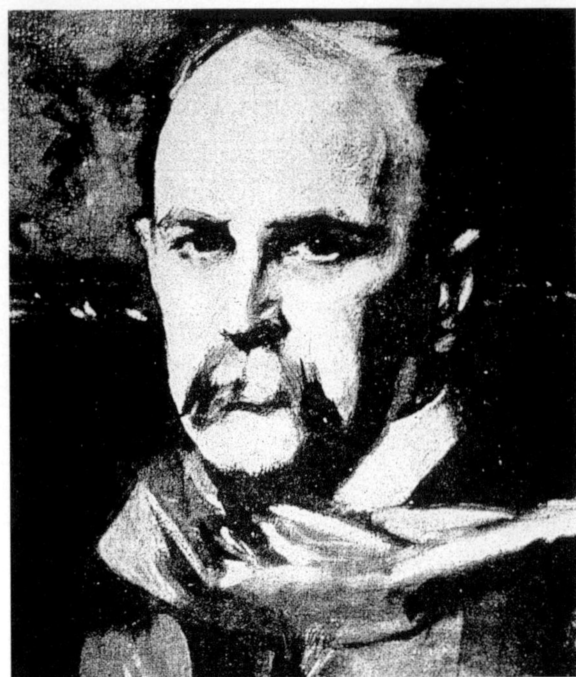

**Figure 1.28** Sir William Osler (1849–1919), Professor of Medicine at Johns Hopkins University, who in his classic textbook *The Principles and Practice of Medicine* (first edition 1892) opined that what we now call 'tension-type headache' was due to 'muscular rheumatism' of the scalp and neck. He called them 'indurative headaches'. The first to hypothesize the existence of 'muscle contraction headaches'

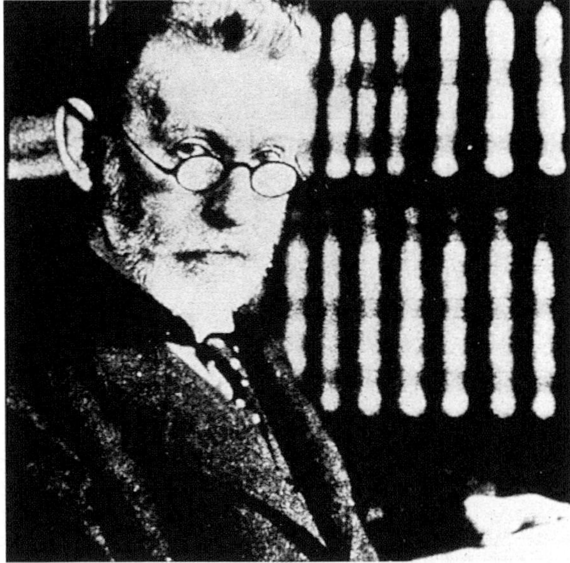

**Figure 1.29** Paul Ehrlich (1854–1915), Nobel Prize winner in 1908, for work on immunology and receptors. Courtesy of the National Library of Medicine, Bethesda, USA

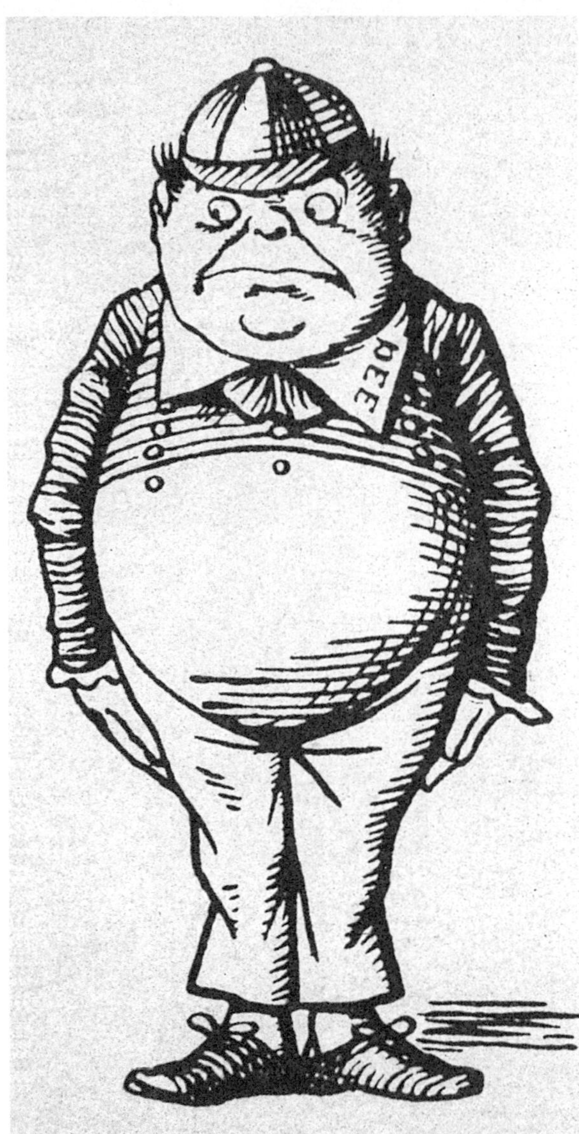


**Figure 1.30** This is Tweedledee, famous for his statement: 'Generally I'm very brave, only today I happen to have a headache'! A John Tenniel illustration

tonin. Sicuteri[16] helped develop methysergide, a serotonin antagonist, for the prophylactic treatment of migraine and cluster headache. After a long hiatus, new drugs are being tested and developed for the preventive treatment of migraine. The anti-epileptic drugs have been investigated and some have already been proven to be effective for migraine. Concomitant with the development of new treatments is the development of the basic sciences of headache and the renewed dedication of clinicians to headache treatment and teaching.

Many scientists, clinicians, and famous migraine sufferers are pictured in the atlas. Artists and advertisers have used their skills to illustrate and illuminate headache, and these illustrations are included.

## REFERENCES


1. Lyons A, Petrucelli RJ. *Medicine: An Illustrated History*. New York: Harry N. Abrams, Inc, 1978:113–5
2. Venzmer G. *Five Thousand Years of Medicine*. New York: Taplinger Publishing Co, 1972:19
3. Rawlings CE, Rossitch E. The history of trepanation in Africa with a discussion of its current status and continuing practice. *Surg Neurol* 1994;41:507–13
4. Critchley M. Migraine: From Cappadocia to Queen Square. In: Smith R, ed. *Background to Migraine*, Volume 1. London: Heinemann, 1967
5. Edmeads J. The treatment of headache: a historical perspective. In: Gallagher RM, ed. *Therapy for Headache*. New York: Marcel Dekker Inc, 1990:1–8
6. Lance JW. *Mechanisms and Management of Headache*, 4th edn. London: Butterworth Scientific, 1982:1–6
7. Singer C. The visions of Hildegarde of Bingen. In: Anonymous. *From Magic to Science*. New York: Dover, 1958
8. Sacks O. *Migraine: Understanding a Common Disorder*. Berkeley: University of California Press, 1985:158–9
9. Patterson SM, Silberstein SD. Sometimes Jello helps: perceptions of headache etiology, triggers and treatment in literature. *Headache* 1993;33:76–81
10. Raskin NH. Migraine: clinical aspects. In: *Headache*, 2nd edn. New York: Churchill-Livingstone, 1988: 35–98
11. Bové FJ. *The Story of Ergot*. New York: Karger, 1970
12. Woakes E. On ergot of rye in the treatment of neuralgia. *Br Med J* 1868;2:360–1
13. Silberstein SD. The pharmacology of ergotamine and dihydroergotamine. *Headache* 1997;37:S15–S25
14. Graham JR, Wolff HG. Mechanisms of migraine headache and action of ergotamine tartrate. *Arch Neurol Psychiatry* 1938;39:737–63
15. Humphrey PP, Feniuk W, Marriott AS, *et al.* Preclinical studies on the anti-migraine drug, sumatriptan. *Eur Neurol* 1991;31:282–90
16. Sicuteri F. Prophylactic and therapeutic properties of 1-methyl-lysergic acid butanolamide in migraine. *Int Arch Allergy* 1959;15:300–7

## FAMOUS MIGRAINE SUFFERERS

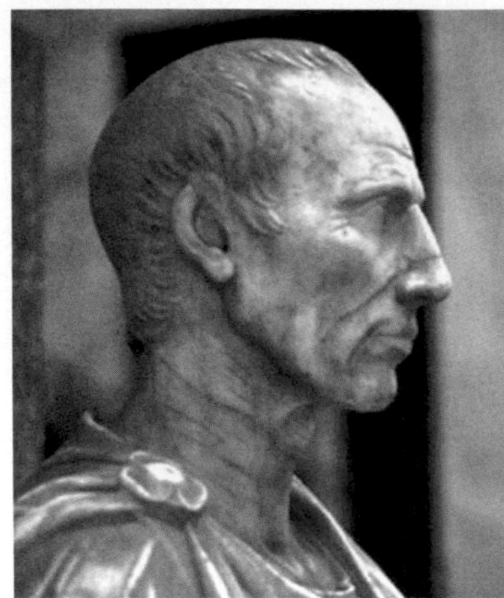

**Julius Caesar 42 BC – AD 37**
Bust from the Vatican museum

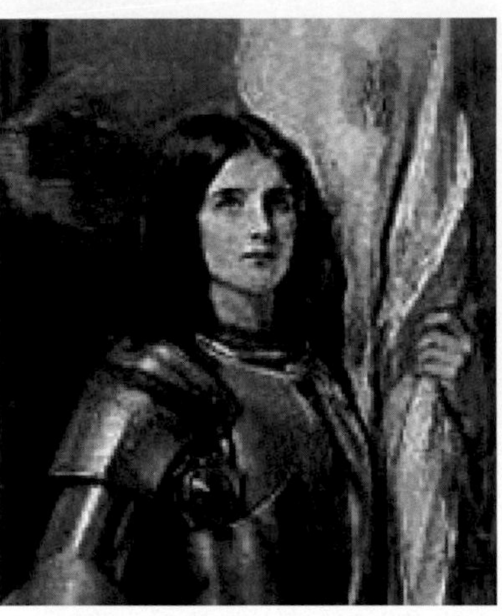

**Joan of Arc 1412–1431**
From Haggard, Andrew C.P. *The France of Joan of Arc*. New York: John Lane Company 1912

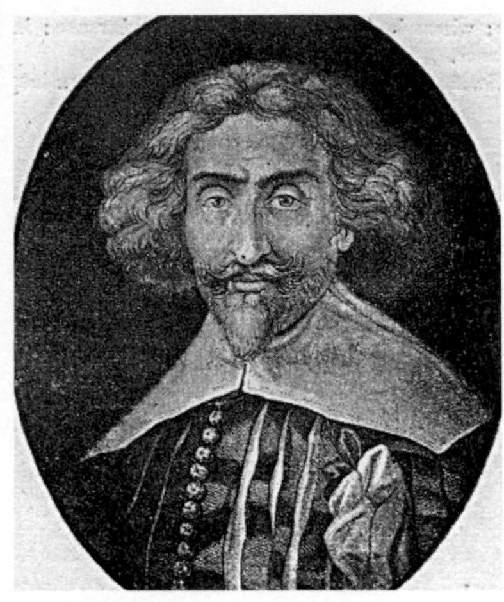

**Miguel de Cervantes Saavedra 1547–1616**
From *The Hundred Greatest Men*. New York: D. Appleton and Company, 1885

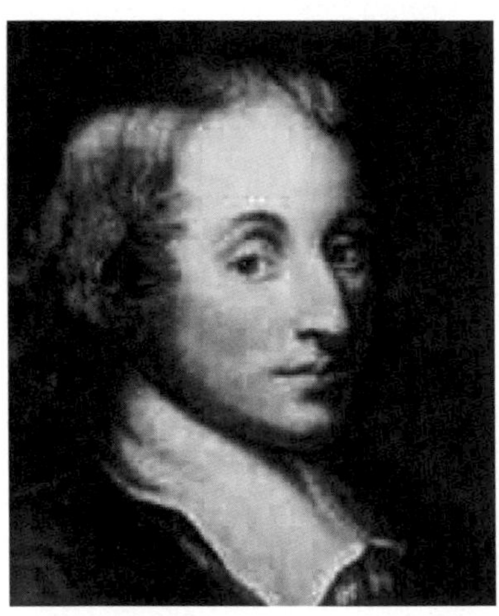

**Blaise Pascal 1623–1662**
Courtesy of web address: http://www.afl.hitos.no/mahist/krydder/pascall.jpg

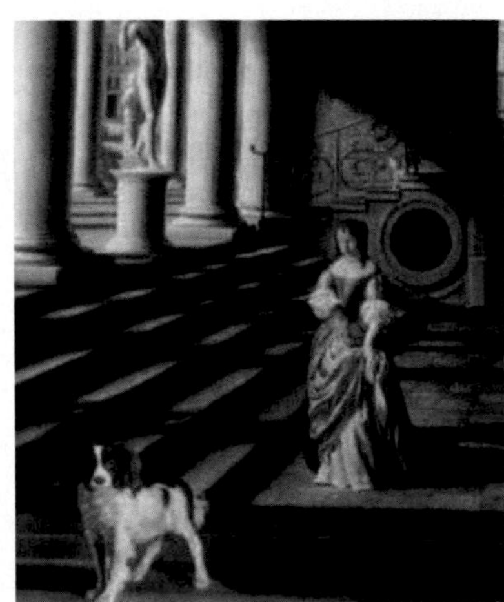

**Anne, Countess of Conway 1631–1679**
With kind permission of Mauritshuis

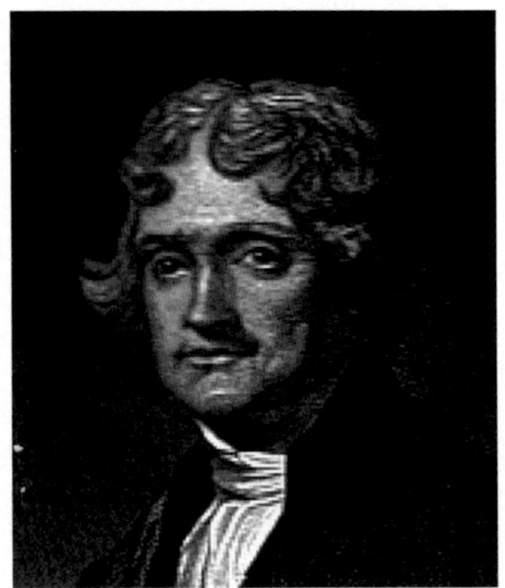

**Thomas Jefferson 1743–1826**
From Duyckinck Evert A. *Portrait Gallery of Eminent Men and Women in Europe and America*. New York: Johnson, Wilson and Company, 1873

## FAMOUS MIGRAINE SUFFERERS

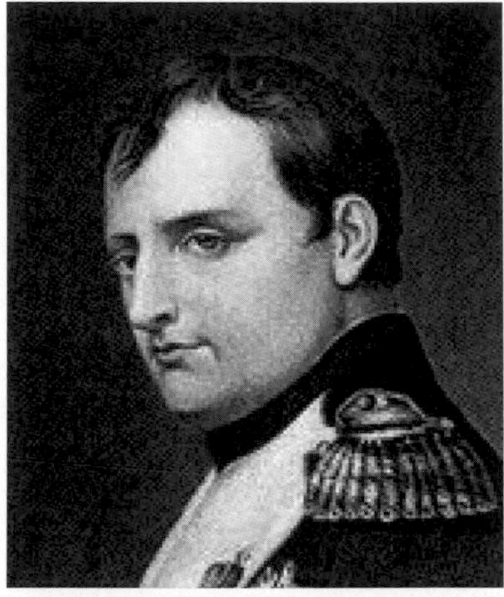

**Napoleon I 1769–1821**
From Duyckinck Evert A. *Portrait Gallery of Eminent Men and Women in Europe and America*. New York: Johnson, Wilson and Company, 1873

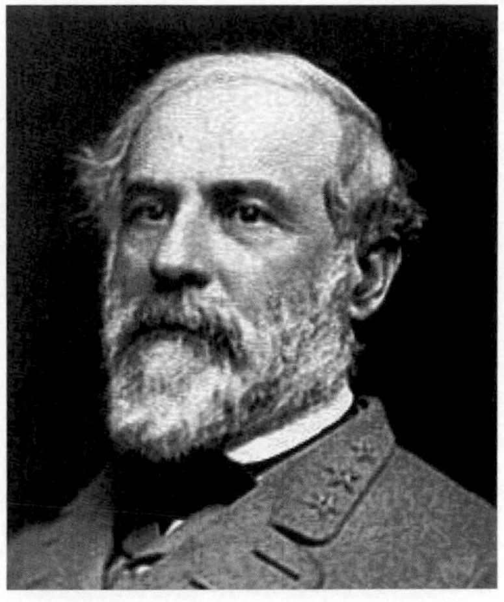

**Robert E. Lee 1807–1870**
Courtesy of the Library of Congress, Prints and Photographs Division, Washington DC 20540, USA (reproduction number, LC-B8172-0001)

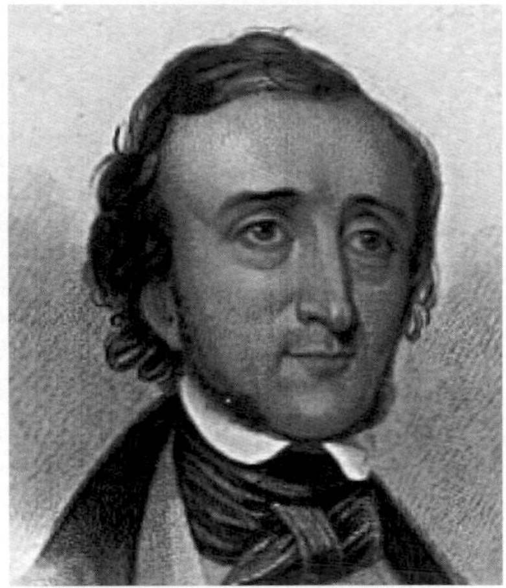

**Edgar Allen Poe 1809–1849**
From Buttre, Lillian C. American Portrait Gallery. New York: J.C. Buttre, 1877

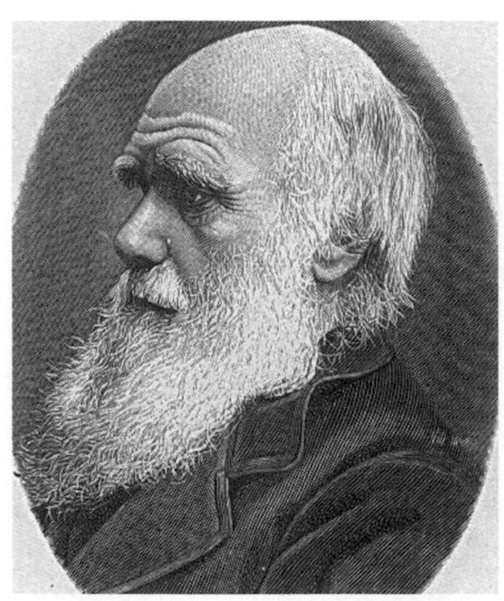

**Charles Darwin 1809–1882**
From Helmot H.F., ed. *History of the World*. New York: Dodd, Mead and Company, 1902

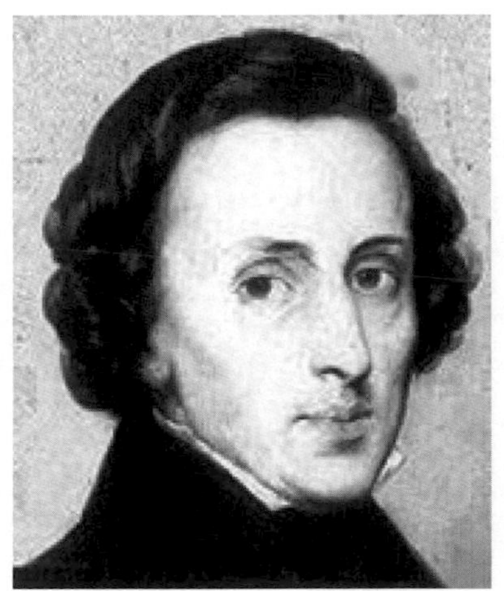

**Frédéric Chopin 1810–1849**
Courtesy of web address: http://inkpot.com/classical/people/chopin3.jpg

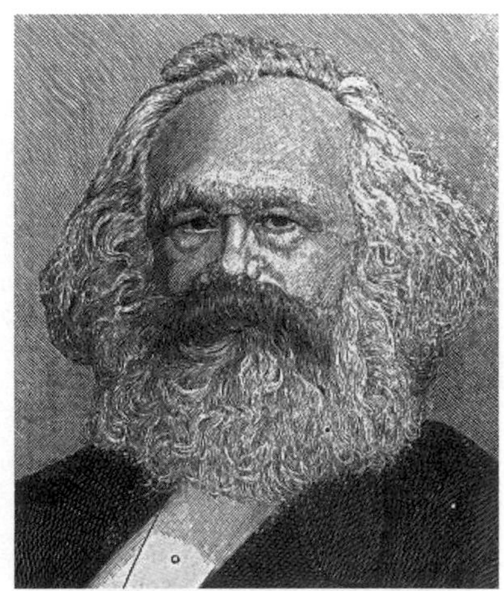

**Karl Marx 1818–1883**
From Helmolt H.F., ed. *History of the World*. New York: Dodd, Mead and Company, 1902

## FAMOUS MIGRAINE SUFFERERS

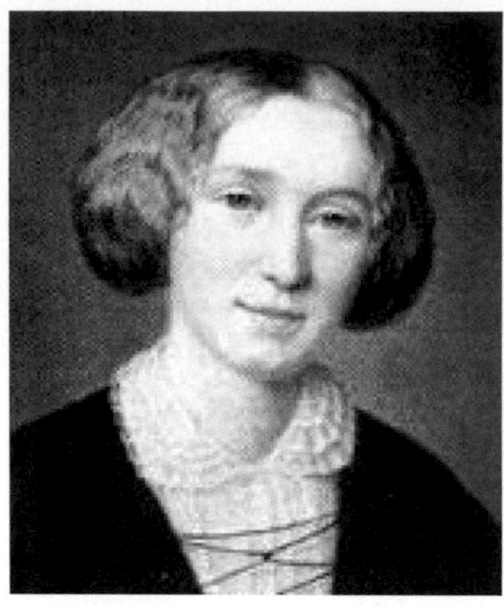

**George Eliot (Mary Ann Evans) 1819–1880**
by A.L. Francois d'Albert-Durade (1804–1886) painted in 1850. With kind permission of The Herbert Art Gallery and Museum, Coventry

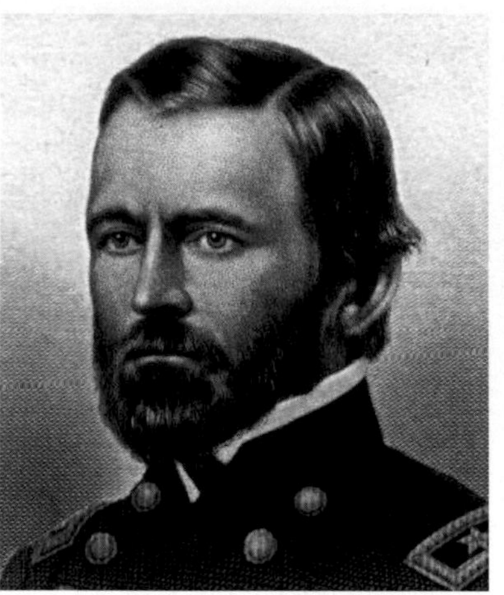

**Ulysses S. Grant 1822–1885**
From Moore F, ed. *Portrait Gallery of the War*. New York: D. van Nostrand, 1865

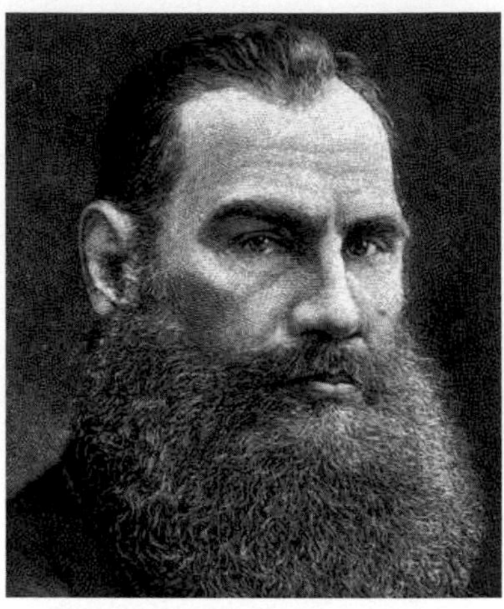

**Leo Tolstoy 1828–1910**
Origin unknown. Produced with kind permission of Leo Finegold, web address: http://www.linguadex.com/tolstoy

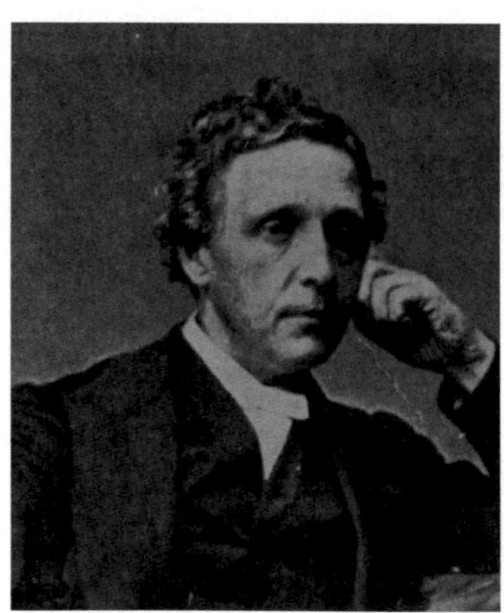

**Lewis Carroll 1832–1898**
Courtesy of the Library of Congress, Prints and Photographs Division, Washington DC 20540, USA (reproduction number, LC-USZ62-70064)

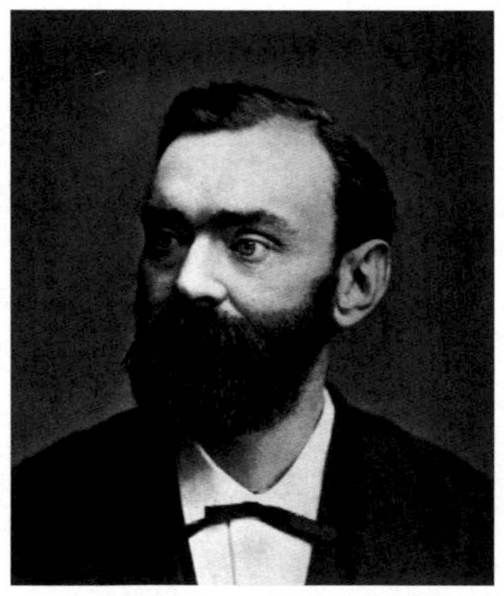

**Alfred Nobel 1833–1896**
With kind permission of © Bettmann/CORBIS

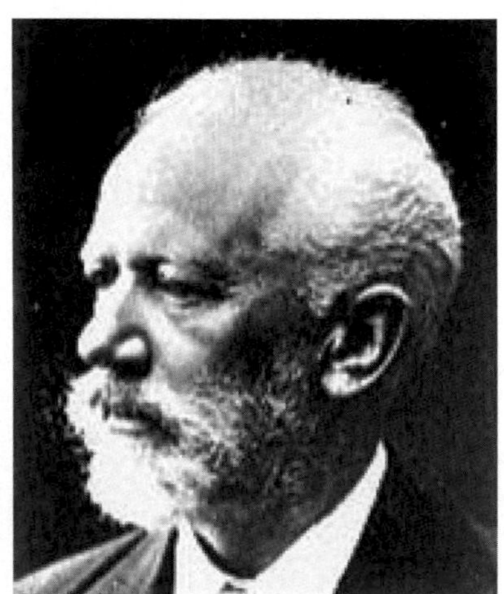

**Pyotyr Ilyich Tchaikovsky 1840–1893**
With kind permission of the Bulfinch's Mythology website: http://www.bulfinch.org

## FAMOUS MIGRAINE SUFFERERS

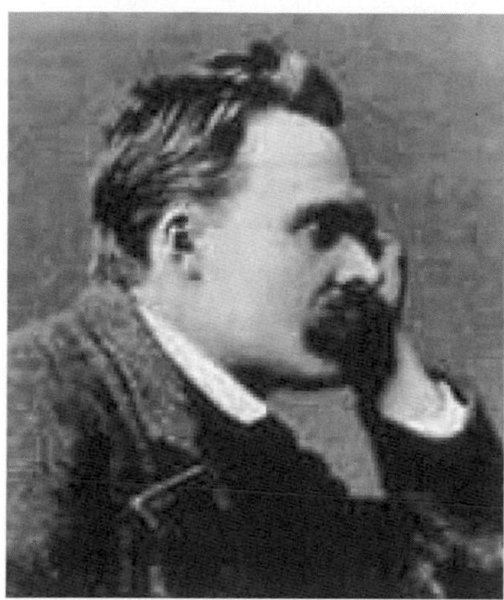

**Friedrich Nietzsche 1844–1900**
Courtesy of web address: http://www.prijatelji-zivotinja.hr/jpg/nietzche.jpg

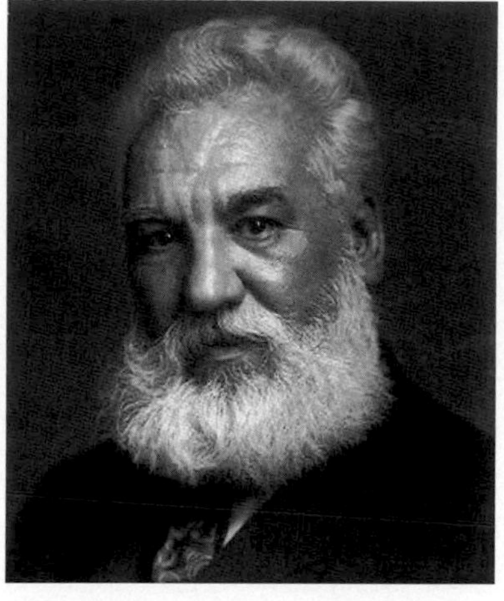

**Alexander Graham Bell 1847–1922**
Courtesy of the Library of Congress, Prints and Photographs Division, Washington DC 20540, USA (reproduction number, LC-USZ62-14759)

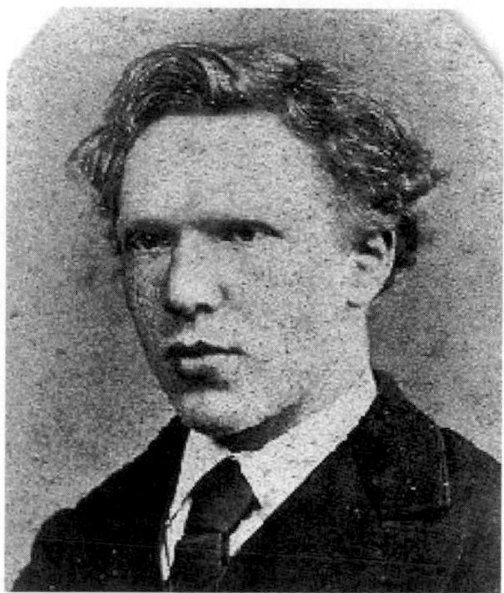

**Vincent van Gogh (aged 19) 1853–1890**
Courtesy of the online Van Gogh Gallery website: http://www.vangoghgallery.com/photos/photo.htm

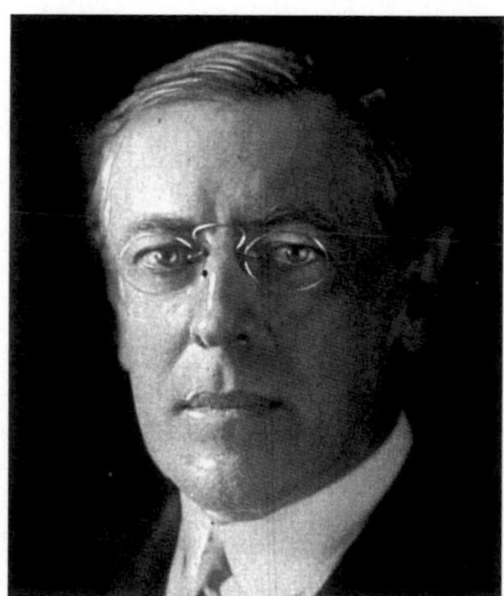

**Thomas Woodrow Wilson 1856–1924**
Courtesy of *Current History of the War* Vol I (December 1914–March 1915). New York: New York Times Company

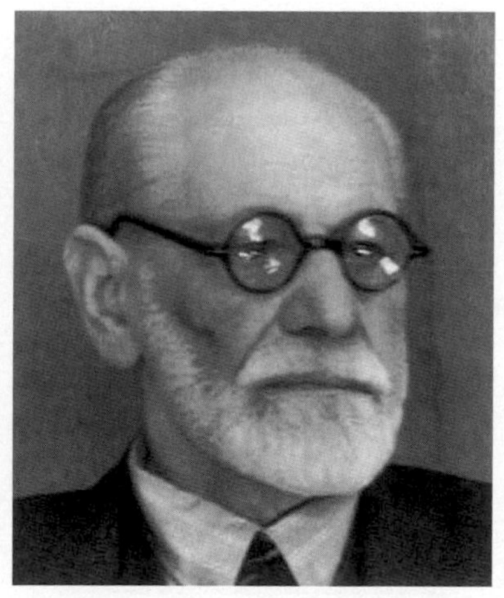

**Sigmund Freud 1856–1939**
Courtesy of the Library of Congress, Prints and Photographs Division, Washington DC 20540, USA (reproduction number, LC-USZ62-72266)

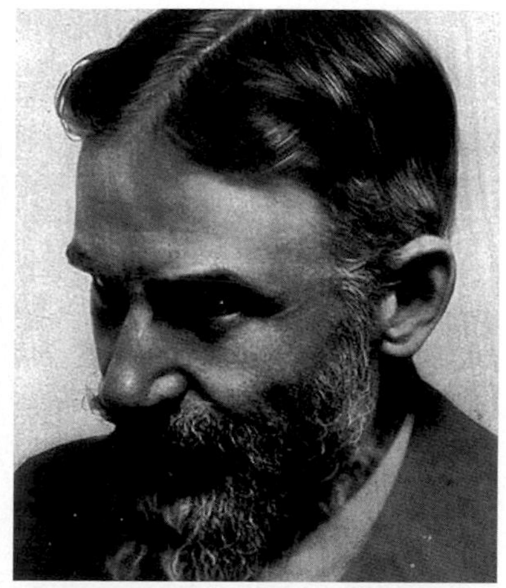

**George Bernard Shaw 1856–1950**
Courtesy of *Current History of the War* Vol I (December 1914–March 1915). New York: New York Times Company

## FAMOUS MIGRAINE SUFFERERS

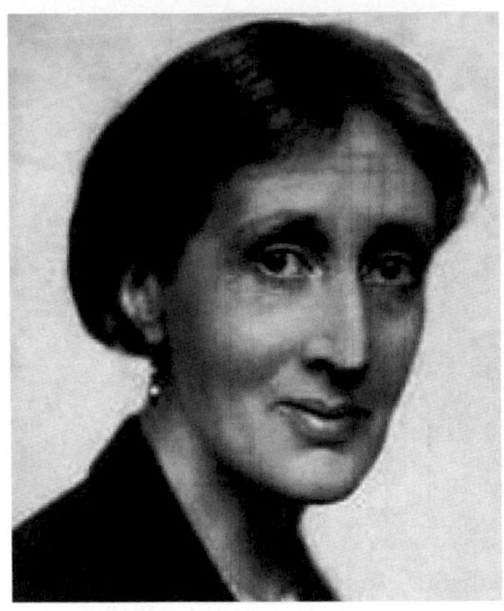

**Virginia Woolf 1882–1941**
Web address:
http://www.marquette.edu/wstudies/woolf-older.jpg

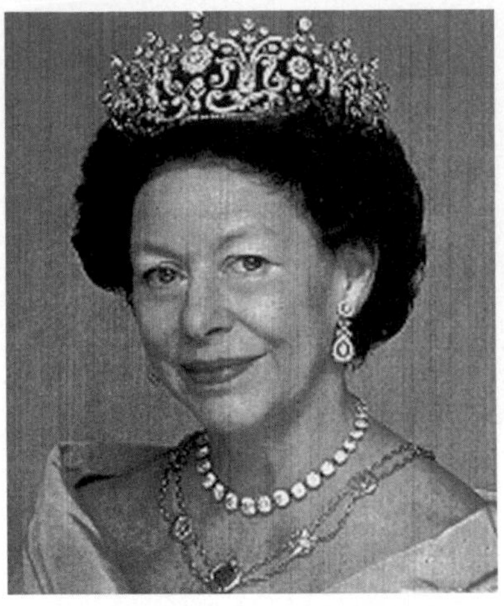

**HRH Princess Margaret 1930–2002**
With kind permission of The Monarchist League of Canada, web address:
http://www.monarchist.ca/margarethello2.jpeg

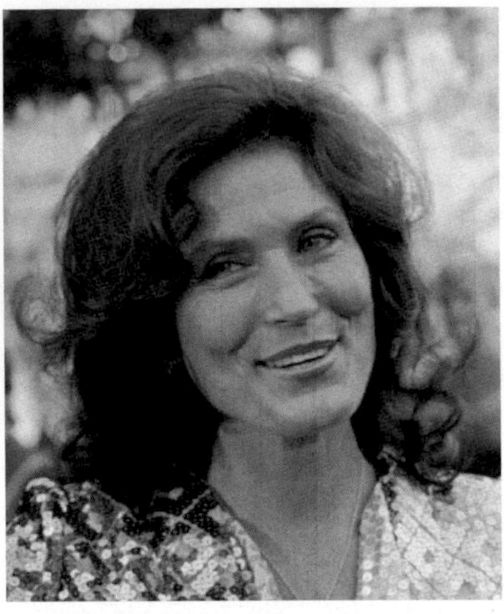

**Loretta Lynn 1934–**
With kind permission of © Bettmann/CORBIS

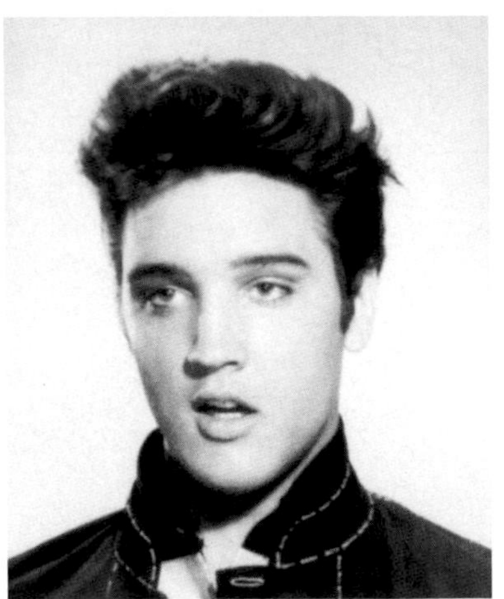

**Elvis Presley 1935–1977**
Courtesy of the Library of Congress, Prints and Photographs Division, Washington D.C. 20540 USA (reproduction number, LC-USZ6-2067)

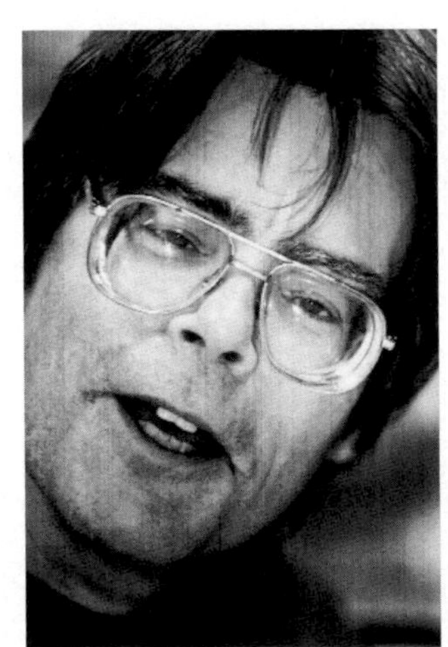

**Stephen King 1947–**
With kind permission of © Rune Hellestad/CORBIS

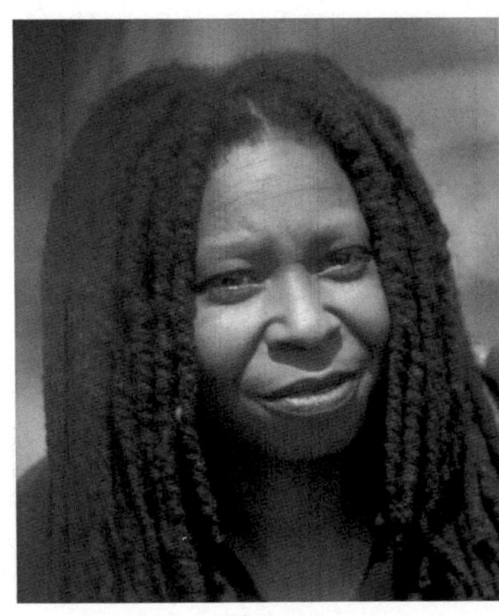

**Whoopi Goldberg 1955–**
With kind permission of © Mitchell Gerber/CORBIS

## FAMOUS MIGRAINE SUFFERERS

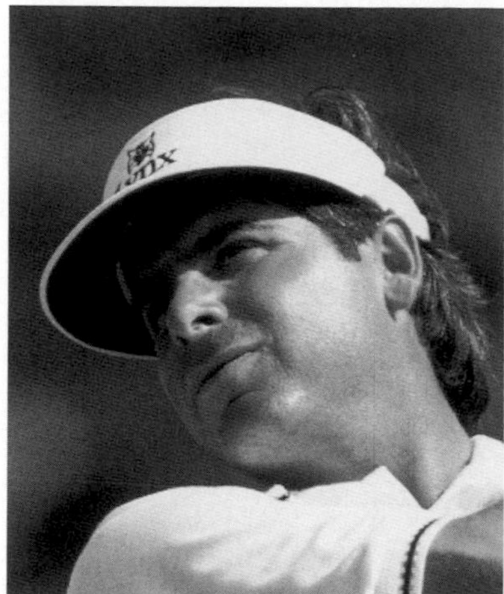

**Fred Couples 1959–**
With kind permission of © Tony Roberts/ CORBIS

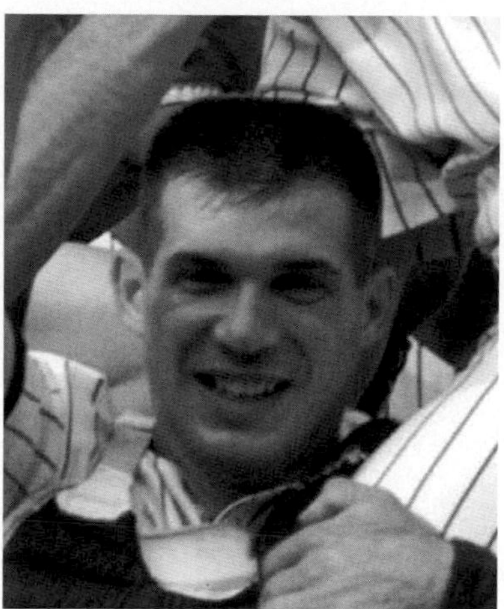

**Joe Girardi 1964–**
With kind permission of © Reuters/CORBIS

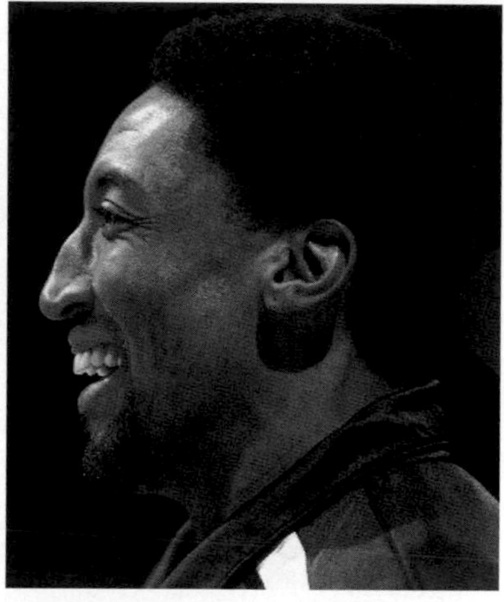

**Scottie Pippin 1965–**
With kind permission of © Greg Fiume/ NewSport/CORBIS

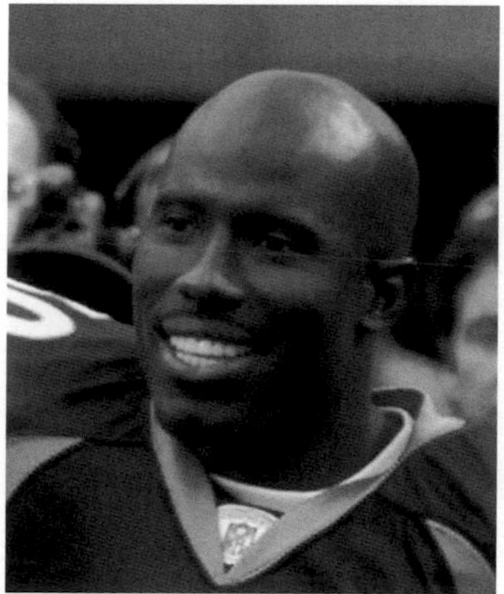

**Terrell Davis 1972–**
With kind permission of © Reuters/CORBIS

# 2

# Headache classification

Elizabeth W Loder

Accurate headache diagnosis is important because it has specific treatment implications. At present, headache diagnosis is clinical; no 'gold standard' tests or biologic markers exist. A widely used classification system is therefore especially important to describe the classic presentation of each headache type and allow study of homogeneous populations of headache sufferers in clinical and scientific trials. The most widely used headache classification system was developed in 1988 by the International Headache Society (IHS), and revised in 2004[1]. In this scheme, headaches are classified using principles similar to those developed by the American Psychiatric Association for psychiatric diagnosis, and assigned to 14 major categories (Table 2.1).

The criteria broadly divide headache into 'primary' and 'secondary' headache disorders.

The primary headache disorders are those in which the headache condition itself is the problem, and no underlying or dangerous cause for it can be identified. The classification is based on symptom profiles. Secondary headaches are those due to an underlying condition such as a tumor, infection or hemorrhage. The secondary headaches are classified according to their causes (e.g. vascular, psychiatric, etc.). Most of the primary and secondary headache disorders are more common in women than in men. Primary headache disorders are much more common than secondary headache disorders.

With the IHS system, each type of headache must be diagnosed and coded, beginning with the patient's most important headache type. When the patient meets all but one of the criteria for a diagnosis, the term *probable* is used. Part 1 of the system classifies the primary headaches, Part 2 classifies the secondary headaches, and Part 3 of the system classifies the cranial neuralgias, central and primary facial pains, and other headaches.

The 'big three' primary headache disorders are migraine, tension-type headaches and cluster headache.

- Migraine is the most common headache problem that causes patients to seek medical help.
- Tension-type headache is the most common headache disorder, but it is usually mild and self-limiting. It generally prompts medical consultation only when chronic.
- Cluster headache is the most severe of the three conditions, but it is uncommon.

## REFERENCE

1. Headache Classification Subcommittee of the International Headache Society. The International Classification of Headache Disorders, 2nd edn. *Cephalalgia* 2004;24(Suppl 1):1–150

**Table 2.1 Classification and WHO ICD-10NA codes**



| IHS ICHD-II code | WHO ICD-10NA code | Diagnosis [and aetiological ICD-10 code for secondary headache disorders] |
|---|---|---|
| **1.** | **[G43]** | **Migraine** |
| 1.1 | [G43.0] | Migraine without aura |
| 1.2 | [G43.1] | Migraine with aura |
| 1.2.1 | [G43.10] | Typical aura with migraine headache |
| 1.2.2 | [G43.10] | Typical aura with non-migraine headache |
| 1.2.3 | [G43.104] | Typical aura without headache |
| 1.2.4 | [G43.105] | Familial hemiplegic migraine (FHM) |
| 1.2.5 | [G43.105] | Sporadic hemiplegic migraine |
| 1.2.6 | [G43.103] | Basilar-type migraine |
| 1.3 | [G43.82] | Childhood periodic syndromes that are commonly precursors of migraine |
| 1.3.1 | [G43.82] | Cyclical vomiting |
| 1.3.2 | [G43.820] | Abdominal migraine |
| 1.3.3 | [G43.821] | Benign paroxysmal vertigo of childhood |
| 1.4 | [G43.81] | Retinal migraine |
| 1.5 | [G43.3] | Complications of migraine |
| 1.5.1 | [G43.3] | Chronic migraine |
| 1.5.2 | [G43.2] | Status migrainosus |
| 1.5.3 | [G43.3] | Persistent aura without infarction |
| 1.5.4 | [G43.3] | Migrainous infarction |
| 1.5.5 | [G43.3] + [G40.x or G41.x][1] | Migraine-triggered seizure |
| 1.6 | [G43.83] | Probable migraine |
| 1.6.1 | [G43.83] | Probable migraine without aura |
| 1.6.2 | [G43.83] | Probable migraine with aura |
| 1.6.3 | [G43.83] | Probable chronic migraine |
| **2.** | **[G44.2]** | **Tension-type headache (TTH)** |
| 2.1 | [G44.2] | Infrequent episodic tension-type headache |
| 2.1.1 | [G44.20] | Infrequent episodic tension-type headache associated with pericranial tenderness |
| 2.1.2 | [G44.21] | Infrequent episodic tension-type headache not associated with pericranial tenderness |
| 2.2 | [G44.2] | Frequent episodic tension-type headache |
| 2.2.1 | [G44.20] | Frequent episodic tension-type headache associated with pericranial tenderness |
| 2.2.2 | [G44.21] | Frequent episodic tension-type headache not associated with pericranial tenderness |
| 2.3 | [G44.2] | Chronic tension-type headache |
| 2.3.1 | [G44.22] | Chronic tension-type headache associated with pericranial tenderness |
| 2.3.2 | [G44.23] | Chronic tension-type headache not associated with pericranial tenderness |
| 2.4 | [G44.28] | Probable tension-type headache |
| 2.4.1 | [G44.28] | Probable infrequent episodic tension-type headache |

[1] The additional code specifies the type of seizure.

**Table 2.1** *continued*

| | | |
|---|---|---|
| 2.4.2 | [G44.28] | Probable frequent episodic tension-type headache |
| 2.4.3 | [G44.28] | Probable chronic tension-type headache |
| **3.** | **[G44.0]** | **Cluster headache and other trigeminal autonomic cephalalgias** |
| 3.1 | [G44.0] | Cluster headache |
| 3.1.1 | [G44.01] | Episodic cluster headache |
| 3.1.2 | [G44.02] | Chronic cluster headache |
| 3.2 | [G44.03] | Paroxysmal hemicrania |
| 3.2.1 | [G44.03] | Episodic paroxysmal hemicrania |
| 3.2.2 | [G44.03] | Chronic paroxysmal hemicrania (CPH) |
| 3.3 | [G44.08] | Short-lasting Unilateral Neuralgiform headache attacks with Conjunctival injection and Tearing (SUNCT) |
| 3.4 | [G44.08] | Probable trigeminal autonomic cephalalgia |
| 3.4.1 | [G44.08] | Probable cluster headache |
| 3.4.2 | [G44.08] | Probable paroxysmal hemicrania |
| 3.4.3 | [G44.08] | Probable SUNCT |
| **4.** | **[G44.80]** | **Other primary headaches** |
| 4.1 | [G44.800] | Primary stabbing headache |
| 4.2 | [G44.803] | Primary cough headache |
| 4.3 | [G44.804] | Primary exertional headache |
| 4.4 | [G44.805] | Primary headache associated with sexual activity |
| 4.4.1 | [G44.805] | Preorgasmic headache |
| 4.4.2 | [G44.805] | Orgasmic headache |
| 4.5 | [G44.80] | Hypnic headache |
| 4.6 | [G44.80] | Primary thunderclap headache |
| 4.7 | [G44.80] | Hemicrania continua |
| 4.8 | [G44.2] | New daily-persistent headache (NDPH) |
| **5.** | **[G44.88]** | **Headache attributed to head and/or neck trauma** |
| 5.1 | [G44.880] | Acute post-traumatic headache |
| 5.1.1 | [G44.880] | Acute post-traumatic headache attributed to moderate or severe head injury [S06] |
| 5.1.2 | [G44.880] | Acute post-traumatic headache attributed to mild head injury [S09.9] |
| 5.2 | [G44.3] | Chronic post-traumatic headache |
| 5.2.1 | [G44.30] | Chronic post-traumatic headache attributed to moderate or severe head injury [S06] |
| 5.2.2 | [G44.31] | Chronic post-traumatic headache attributed to mild head injury [S09.9] |
| 5.3 | [G44.841] | Acute headache attributed to whiplash injury [S13.4] |
| 5.4 | [G44.841] | Chronic headache attributed to whiplash injury [S13.4] |
| 5.5 | [G44.88] | Headache attributed to traumatic intracranial haematoma |
| 5.5.1 | [G44.88] | Headache attributed to epidural haematoma [S06.4] |
| 5.5.2 | [G44.88] | Headache attributed to subdural haematoma [S06.5] |
| 5.6 | [G44.88] | Headache attributed to other head and/or neck trauma [S06] |
| 5.6.1 | [G44.88] | Acute headache attributed to other head and/or neck trauma [S06] |
| 5.6.2 | [G44.88] | Chronic headache attributed to other head and/or neck trauma [S06] |
| 5.7 | [G44.88] | Post-craniotomy headache |
| 5.7.1 | [G44.880] | Acute post-craniotomy headache |
| 5.7.2 | [G44.30] | Chronic post-craniotomy headache |
| **6.** | **[G44.81]** | **Headache attributed to cranial or cervical vascular disorder** |
| 6.1 | [G44.810] | Headache attributed to ischaemic stroke or transient ischaemic attack |
| 6.1.1 | [G44.810] | Headache attributed to ischaemic stroke (cerebral infarction) [I63] |
| 6.1.2 | [G44.810] | Headache attributed to transient ischaemic attack (TIA) [G45] |

**Table 2.1** *continued*

| | | |
|---|---|---|
| 6.2 | [G44.810] | Headache attributed to non-traumatic intracranial haemorrhage [I62] |
| 6.2.1 | [G44.810] | Headache attributed to intracerebral haemorrhage [I61] |
| 6.2.2 | [G44.810] | Headache attributed to subarachnoid haemorrhage (SAH) [I60] |
| 6.3 | [G44.811] | Headache attributed to unruptured vascular malformation [Q28] |
| 6.3.1 | [G44.811] | Headache attributed to saccular aneurysm [Q28.3] |
| 6.3.2 | [G44.811] | Headache attributed to arteriovenous malformation (AVM) [Q28.2] |
| 6.3.3 | [G44.811] | Headache attributed to dural arteriovenous fistula [I67.1] |
| 6.3.4 | [G44.811] | Headache attributed to cavernous angioma [D18.0] |
| 6.3.5 | [G44.811] | Headache attributed to encephalotrigeminal or leptomeningeal angiomatosis (Sturge Weber syndrome) [Q85.8] |
| 6.4 | [G44.812] | Headache attributed to arteritis [M31] |
| 6.4.1 | [G44.812] | Headache attributed to giant cell arteritis (GCA) [M31.6] |
| 6.4.2 | [G44.812] | Headache attributed to primary central nervous system (CNS) angiitis [I67.7] |
| 6.4.3 | [G44.812] | Headache attributed to secondary central nervous system (CNS) angiitis [I68.2] |
| 6.5 | [G44.810] | Carotid or vertebral artery pain [I63.0, I63.2, I65.0, I65.2 or I67.0] |
| 6.5.1 | [G44.810] | Headache or facial or neck pain attributed to arterial dissection [I67.0] |
| 6.5.2 | [G44.814] | Post-endarterectomy headache [I97.8] |
| 6.5.3 | [G44.810] | Carotid angioplasty headache |
| 6.5.4 | [G44.810] | Headache attributed to intracranial endovascular procedures |
| 6.5.5 | [G44.810] | Angiography headache |
| 6.6 | [G44.810] | Headache attributed to cerebral venous thrombosis (CVT) [I63.6] |
| 6.7 | [G44.81] | Headache attributed to other intracranial vascular disorder |
| 6.7.1 | [G44.81] | Cerebral Autosomal Dominant Arteriopathy with Subcortical Infarcts and Leukoencephalopathy (CADASIL) [I67.8] |
| 6.7.2 | [G44.81] | Mitochondrial Encephalopathy, Lactic Acidosis and Stroke-like episodes (MELAS) [G31.81] |
| 6.7.3 | [G44.81] | Headache attributed to benign angiopathy of the central nervous system [I99] |
| 6.7.4 | [G44.81] | Headache attributed to pituitary apoplexy [E23.6] |
| **7.** | **[G44.82]** | **Headache attributed to non-vascular intracranial disorder** |
| 7.1 | [G44.820] | Headache attributed to high cerebrospinal fluid pressure |
| 7.1.1 | [G44.820] | Headache attributed to idiopathic intracranial hypertension (IIH) [G93.2] |
| 7.1.2 | [G44.820] | Headache attributed to intracranial hypertension secondary to metabolic, toxic or hormonal causes |
| 7.1.3 | [G44.820] | Headache attributed to intracranial hypertension secondary to hydrocephalus [G91.8] |
| 7.2 | [G44.820] | Headache attributed to low cerebrospinal fluid pressure |
| 7.2.1 | [G44.820] | Post-dural puncture headache [G97.0] |
| 7.2.2 | [G44.820] | CSF fistula headache [G96.0] |
| 7.2.3 | [G44.820] | Headache attributed to spontaneous (or idiopathic) low CSF pressure |
| 7.3 | [G44.82] | Headache attributed to non-infectious inflammatory disease |
| 7.3.1 | [G44.823] | Headache attributed to neurosarcoidosis [D86.8] |
| 7.3.2 | [G44.823] | Headache attributed to aseptic (non-infectious) meningitis [code to specify aetiology] |
| 7.3.3 | [G44.823] | Headache attributed to other non-infectious inflammatory disease [code to specify aetiology] |
| 7.3.4 | [G44.82] | Headache attributed to lymphocytic hypophysitis [E23.6] |
| 7.4 | [G44.822] | Headache attributed to intracranial neoplasm [C00-D48] |
| 7.4.1 | [G44.822] | Headache attributed to increased intracranial pressure or hydrocephalus caused by neoplasm [code to specify neoplasm] |

**Table 2.1** *continued*

| | | |
|---|---|---|
| 7.4.2 | [G44.822] | Headache attributed directly to neoplasm [code to specify neoplasm] |
| 7.4.3 | [G44.822] | Headache attributed to carcinomatous meningitis [C79.3] |
| 7.4.4 | [G44.822] | Headache attributed to hypothalamic or pituitary hyper- or hyposecretion [E23.0] |
| 7.5 | [G44.824] | Headache attributed to intrathecal injection [G97.8] |
| 7.6 | [G44.82] | Headache attributed to epileptic seizure [G40.x or G41.x to specify seizure type] |
| 7.6.1 | [G44.82] | Hemicrania epileptica [G40.x or G41.x to specify seizure type] |
| 7.6.2 | [G44.82] | Post-seizure headache [G40.x or G41.x to specify seizure type] |
| 7.7 | [G44.82] | Headache attributed to Chiari malformation type I (CM1) [Q07.0] |
| 7.8 | [G44.82] | Syndrome of transient Headache and Neurological Deficits with cerebrospinal fluid Lymphocytosis (HaNDL) |
| 7.9 | [G44.82] | Headache attributed to other non-vascular intracranial disorder |
| **8.** | **[G44.4 or G44.83]** | **Headache attributed to a substance[2] or its withdrawal** |
| 8.1 | [G44.40] | Headache induced by acute substance use or exposure |
| 8.1.1 | [G44.400] | Nitric oxide (NO) donor-induced headache [X44] |
| 8.1.1.1 | [G44.400] | Immediate NO donor-induced headache [X44] |
| 8.1.1.2 | [G44.400] | Delayed NO donor-headache [X44] |
| 8.1.2 | [G44.40] | Phosphodiesterase (PDE) inhibitor-induced headache [X44] |
| 8.1.3 | [G44.402] | Carbon monoxide-induced headache [X47] |
| 8.1.4 | [G44.83] | Alcohol-induced headache [F10] |
| 8.1.4.1 | [G44.83] | Immediate alcohol-induced headache [F10] |
| 8.1.4.2 | [G44.83] | Delayed alcohol-induced headache [F10] |
| 8.1.5 | [G44.4] | Headache induced by food components and additives |
| 8.1.5.1 | [G44.401] | Monosodium glutamate-induced headache [X44] |
| 8.1.6 | [G44.83] | Cocaine-induced headache [F14] |
| 8.1.7 | [G44.83] | Cannabis-induced headache [F12] |
| 8.1.8 | [G44.40] | Histamine-induced headache [X44] |
| 8.1.8.1 | [G44.40] | Immediate histamine-induced headache [X44] |
| 8.1.8.2 | [G44.40] | Delayed histamine-induced headache [X44] |
| 8.1.9 | [G44.40] | Calcitonin gene-related peptide (CGRP)-induced headache [X44] |
| 8.1.9.1 | [G44.40] | Immediate CGRP-induced headache [X44] |
| 8.1.9.2 | [G44.40] | Delayed CGRP-induced headache [X44] |
| 8.1.10 | [G44.41] | Headache as an acute adverse event attributed to medication used for other indications [code to specify substance] |
| 8.1.11 | [G44.4 or G44.83] | Headache induced by other acute substance use or exposure [code to specify substance] |
| 8.2 | [G44.41 or G44.83] | Medication-overuse headache (MOH) |
| 8.2.1 | [G44.411] | Ergotamine-overuse headache [Y52.5] |
| 8.2.2 | [G44.41] | Triptan-overuse headache |
| 8.2.3 | [G44.410] | Analgesic-overuse headache [F55.2] |
| 8.2.4 | [G44.83] | Opioid-overuse headache [F11.2] |
| 8.2.5 | [G44.410] | Combination medication-overuse headache [F55.2] |
| 8.2.6 | [G44.410] | Headache attributed to other medication overuse [code to specify substance] |
| 8.2.7 | [G44.41 or G44.83] | Probable medication-overuse headache [code to specify substance] |

[2] In ICD-10 substances are classified according to the presence or absence of a dependence-producing property. Headaches associated with psychoactive substances (dependence-producing) are classified in G44.83 with an additional code to indicate the nature of the disorder related to the substance use: *eg*, intoxication (F1x.0), dependence (F1x.2), withdrawal (F1x.3), *etc.* The 3rd character can be used to indicate the specific substance involved: *eg*, F10 for alcohol, F15 for caffeine, *etc.* Abuse of non-dependence-producing substances is classified in F55, with a 4th character to indicate the substance: *eg*, F55.2 abuse of analgesics. Headaches related to non-dependence-producing substances are classified in G44.4.

**Table 2.1** *continued*

| | | |
|---|---|---|
| 8.3 | [G44.4] | Headache as an adverse event attributed to chronic medication [code to specify substance] |
| 8.3.1 | [G44.418] | Exogenous hormone-induced headache [Y42.4] |
| 8.4 | [G44.83] | Headache attributed to substance withdrawal |
| 8.4.1 | [G44.83] | Caffeine-withdrawal headache [F15.3] |
| 8.4.2 | [G44.83] | Opioid-withdrawal headache [F11.3] |
| 8.4.3 | [G44.83] | Oestrogen-withdrawal headache [Y42.4] |
| 8.4.4 | [G44.83] | Headache attributed to withdrawal from chronic use of other substances [code to specify substance] |
| **9.** | | **Headache attributed to infection** |
| 9.1 | [G44.821] | Headache attributed to intracranial infection [G00-G09] |
| 9.1.1 | [G44.821] | Headache attributed to bacterial meningitis [G00.9] |
| 9.1.2 | [G44.821] | Headache attributed to lymphocytic meningitis [G03.9] |
| 9.1.3 | [G44.821] | Headache attributed to encephalitis [G04.9] |
| 9.1.4 | [G44.821] | Headache attributed to brain abscess [G06.0] |
| 9.1.5 | [G44.821] | Headache attributed to subdural empyema [G06.2] |
| 9.2 | [G44.881] | Headache attributed to systemic infection [A00-B97] |
| 9.2.1 | [G44.881] | Headache attributed to systemic bacterial infection [code to specify aetiology] |
| 9.2.2 | [G44.881] | Headache attributed to systemic viral infection [code to specify aetiology] |
| 9.2.3 | [G44.881] | Headache attributed to other systemic infection [code to specify aetiology] |
| 9.3 | [G44.821] | Headache attributed to HIV/AIDS [B22] |
| 9.4 | [G44.821 or G44.881] | Chronic post-infection headache [code to specify aetiology] |
| 9.4.1 | [G44.821] | Chronic post-bacterial meningitis headache [G00.9] |
| **10.** | **[G44.882]** | **Headache attributed to disorder of homoeostasis** |
| 10.1 | [G44.882] | Headache attributed to hypoxia and/or hypercapnia |
| 10.1.1 | [G44.882] | High-altitude headache [W94] |
| 10.1.2 | [G44.882] | Diving headache |
| 10.1.3 | [G44.882] | Sleep apnoea headache [G47.3] |
| 10.2 | [G44.882] | Dialysis headache [Y84.1] |
| 10.3 | [G44.813] | Headache attributed to arterial hypertension [I10] |
| 10.3.1 | [G44.813] | Headache attributed to phaeochromocytoma [D35.0 (benign) or C74.1 (malignant)] |
| 10.3.2 | [G44.813] | Headache attributed to hypertensive crisis without hypertensive encephalopathy [I10] |
| 10.3.3 | [G44.813] | Headache attributed to hypertensive encephalopathy [I67.4] |
| 10.3.4 | [G44.813] | Headache attributed to pre-eclampsia [O13-O14] |
| 10.3.5 | [G44.813] | Headache attributed to eclampsia [O15] |
| 10.3.6 | [G44.813] | Headache attributed to acute pressor response to an exogenous agent [code to specify aetiology] |
| 10.4 | [G44.882] | Headache attributed to hypothyroidism [E03.9] |
| 10.5 | [G44.882] | Headache attributed to fasting [T73.0] |
| 10.6 | [G44.882] | Cardiac cephalalgia [code to specify aetiology] |
| 10.7 | [G44.882] | Headache attributed to other disorder of homoeostasis [code to specify aetiology] |
| **11.** | **[G44.84]** | **Headache or facial pain attributed to disorder of cranium, neck, eyes, ears, nose, sinuses, teeth, mouth or other facial or cranial structures** |
| 11.1 | [G44.840] | Headache attributed to disorder of cranial bone [M80-M89.8] |

**Table 2.1** *continued*

| | | |
|---|---|---|
| 11.2 | [G44.841] | Headache attributed to disorder of neck [M99] |
| 11.2.1 | [G44.841] | Cervicogenic headache [M99] |
| 11.2.2 | [G44.842] | Headache attributed to retropharyngeal tendonitis [M79.8] |
| 11.2.3 | [G44.841] | Headache attributed to craniocervical dystonia [G24] |
| 11.3 | [G44.843] | Headache attributed to disorder of eyes |
| 11.3.1 | [G44.843] | Headache attributed to acute glaucoma [H40] |
| 11.3.2 | [G44.843] | Headache attributed to refractive errors [H52] |
| 11.3.3 | [G44.843] | Headache attributed to heterophoria or heterotropia (latent or manifest squint) [H50.3-H50.5] |
| 11.3.4 | [G44.843] | Headache attributed to ocular inflammatory disorder [code to specify aetiology] |
| 11.4 | [G44.844] | Headache attributed to disorder of ears [H60-H95] |
| 11.5 | [G44.845] | Headache attributed to rhinosinusitis [J01] |
| 11.6 | [G44.846] | Headache attributed to disorder of teeth, jaws or related structures [K00-K14] |
| 11.7 | [G44.846] | Headache or facial pain attributed to temporomandibular joint (TMJ) disorder [K07.6] |
| 11.8 | [G44.84] | Headache attributed to other disorder of cranium, neck, eyes, ears, nose, sinuses, teeth, mouth or other facial or cervical structures [code to specify aetiology] |
| **12.** | **[R51]** | **Headache attributed to psychiatric disorder** |
| 12.1 | [R51] | Headache attributed to somatisation disorder [F45.0] |
| 12.2 | [R51] | Headache attributed to psychotic disorder [code to specify aetiology] |
| **13.** | **[G44.847, G44.848 or G44.85]** | **Cranial neuralgias and central causes of facial pain** |
| 13.1 | [G44.847] | Trigeminal neuralgia |
| 13.1.1 | [G44.847] | Classical trigeminal neuralgia [G50.00] |
| 13.1.2 | [G44.847] | Symptomatic trigeminal neuralgia [G53.80] + [code to specify aetiology] |
| 13.2 | [G44.847] | Glossopharyngeal neuralgia |
| 13.2.1 | [G44.847] | Classical glossopharyngeal neuralgia [G52.10] |
| 13.2.2 | [G44.847] | Symptomatic glossopharyngeal neuralgia [G53.830] + [code to specify aetiology] |
| 13.3 | [G44.847] | Nervus intermedius neuralgia [G51.80] |
| 13.4 | [G44.847] | Superior laryngeal neuralgia [G52.20] |
| 13.5 | [G44.847] | Nasociliary neuralgia [G52.80] |
| 13.6 | [G44.847] | Supraorbital neuralgia [G52.80] |
| 13.7 | [G44.847] | Other terminal branch neuralgias [G52.80] |
| 13.8 | [G44.847] | Occipital neuralgia [G52.80] |
| 13.9 | [G44.851] | Neck-tongue syndrome |
| 13.10 | [G44.801] | External compression headache |
| 13.11 | [G44.802] | Cold-stimulus headache |
| 13.11.1 | [G44.8020] | Headache attributed to external application of a cold stimulus |
| 13.11.2 | [G44.8021] | Headache attributed to ingestion or inhalation of a cold stimulus |
| 13.12 | [G44.848] | Constant pain caused by compression, irritation or distortion of cranial nerves or upper cervical roots by structural lesions [G53.8] + [code to specify aetiology] |
| 13.13 | [G44.848] | Optic neuritis [H46] |
| 13.14 | [G44.848] | Ocular diabetic neuropathy [E10-E14] |
| 13.15 | [G44.881 or G44.847] | Head or facial pain attributed to herpes zoster |
| 13.15.1 | [G44.881] | Head or facial pain attributed to acute herpes zoster [B02.2] |
| 13.15.2 | [G44.847] | Post-herpetic neuralgia [B02.2] |

**Table 2.1** *continued*

| | | |
|---|---|---|
| 13.16 | [G44.850] | Tolosa-Hunt syndrome |
| 13.17 | [G43.80] | Ophthalmoplegic 'migraine' |
| 13.18 | [G44.810 or G44.847] | Central causes of facial pain |
| 13.18.1 | [G44.847] | Anaesthesia dolorosa [G52.800] + [code to specify aetiology] |
| 13.18.2 | [G44.810] | Central post-stroke pain [G46.21] |
| 13.18.3 | [G44.847] | Facial pain attributed to multiple sclerosis [G35] |
| 13.18.4 | [G44.847] | Persistent idiopathic facial pain [G50.1] |
| 13.18.5 | [G44.847] | Burning mouth syndrome [code to specify aetiology] |
| 13.19 | [G44.847] | Other cranial neuralgia or other centrally mediated facial pain [code to specify aetiology] |
| **14.** | **[R51]** | **Other headache, cranial neuralgia, central or primary facial pain** |
| 14.1 | [R51] | Headache not elsewhere classified |
| 14.2 | [R51] | Headache unspecified |

# 3

# Epidemiology of migraine

Mario F P Peres

## INTRODUCTION

Headaches are one of the most common complaints encountered by the practicing physician. Despite the amount of suffering and disability they cause, headaches are still underdiagnosed and undertreated.

Epidemiology has important implications for the diagnosis and treatment of headache disorders. Examination of sociodemographic, distribution, impact, familial and environmental risk factors may provide clues to preventive strategies and disease mechanisms. In this chapter, epidemiologic terms, prevalence rates, impact, costs and comorbidity of migraine are reviewed.

## DEFINITIONS OF EPIDEMIOLOGIC TERMS

For clinical practice and epidemiologic research, it is important to have precise definitions to enable reliable and valid diagnosis (Figure 3.1). Since there is no true diagnostic gold standard for the primary headache disorders, it is difficult to study validity and to define diagnostic boundaries for symptom-based conditions.

Epidemiologic studies often focus on prevalence or incidence. Prevalence is the proportion of a given population that has a disorder over a defined period of time. Lifetime prevalence is the proportion of individuals who have ever had the condition, and one-year prevalence is the proportion of individuals who have had at least one attack within one year. Incidence is the onset of new cases of a disease in a defined population over a given period of time.

## EPIDEMIOLOGY OF PRIMARY AND SECONDARY HEADACHES

Using the IHS criteria, Rasmussen *et al.*[1] examined the population distribution of all headache disorders via in-person clinical assessment in a large, representative community sample in the greater Copenhagen area. The lifetime prevalence of tension-type headache was 78% and that of migraine 16%. The most common secondary cause was fasting, which was the case in 19% of patients, followed by nose/sinus disease in 15% of patients and head trauma in 4%. Non-vascular intracranial disease, including brain tumor, accounted for 0.5%. Rasmussen and Olesen[2] studied the epidemiology of other headache disorders. Lifetime prevalence of idiopathic stabbing headache was 2%, external compression headache was 4% and cold stimulus headache was 15%. Benign cough headache, benign exertional headache and headache associated with sexual activity were each 1%. Lifetime prevalence of hangover headache was 72%, of fever headache 63% and of headache associated with disorders of the nose or sinuses 15%. Headaches associated with severe structural lesions were rare. Most headaches showed a significant female predominance. Symptomatic headaches were more prevalent among migraineurs. In subjects with tension-type headache, only hangover headache was over-represented. There was no association between the headache disorders and abnormal routine blood chemistries or arterial hypertension. In women with migraine, however, diastolic blood pressure was significantly higher than in women without migraine.

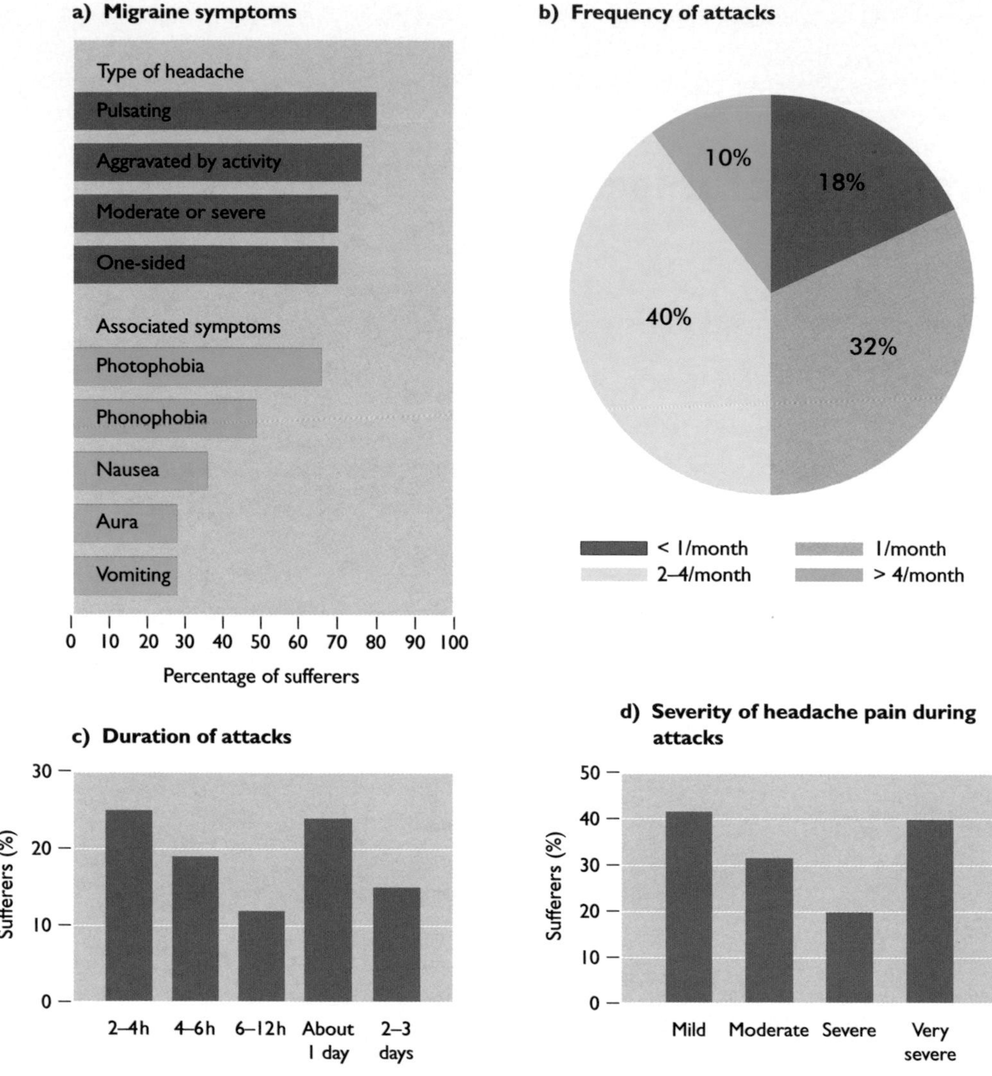


**Figure 3.1** Migraine characteristics from population studies of migraine epidemiology using the diagnostic criteria of the International Headache Society (IHS). (a) Adapted with permission from Micieli G. Suffering in silence. In: Edmeads J, ed. *Migraine: A Brighter Future*, 1993:1–7, with permission of Cambridge Medical Publications; (b) to (d) data derived from Henry P, Michel P, Brochet B, *et al.* A nationwide survey of migraine in France: prevalence and clinical features in adults. *Cephalalgia* 1992;12:229–37

## MIGRAINE

Migraine is a very common condition worldwide. Estimates of its prevalence have varied widely, ranging from 3% to about 22% (Figure 3.2). The differences can be accounted for by the differing definitions and methodologies employed. A reasonable estimate of one-year prevalence of migraine in adults is 10 to 12% (6% in men and 15–18% in women). In a Danish epidemiologic study[3], lifetime prevalence of migraine was 16% (8% in men and 25% in women) and one-year prevalence was 10% (6% in men and 15% in women). Prevalence of migraine without aura was 6% and that of migraine with aura was 4%.

In the US population, the one-year prevalence of migraine was 12% (6% in men and 18% in women)[4]. The same rates were found in France[5]. Migraine has been estimated to affect 1.5% of people in Hong Kong, 2.6% in Saudi Arabia, and 3% in Ethiopia. In

Japan and Malaysia, prevalence rates were similar to those found in Western countries (8.4 and 9.0%, respectively; Figure 3.3). A recent epidemiologic study in South America[6] showed one-year prevalence of migraine in women (men) of 17% (8) in Brazil, 6% (4) in Argentina, 14% (5) in Colombia, 12% (4) in Mexico and 12% (5) in Venezuela.

Migraine prevalence is age- and gender-dependent. Before puberty, migraine is slightly more common in boys, with the highest incidence between 6–10 years of age. In women, the incidence is highest between 14–19 years of age. In general, women are more commonly affected than men (Figure 3.4), with a lifetime prevalence of 12–17% and 4–6%,

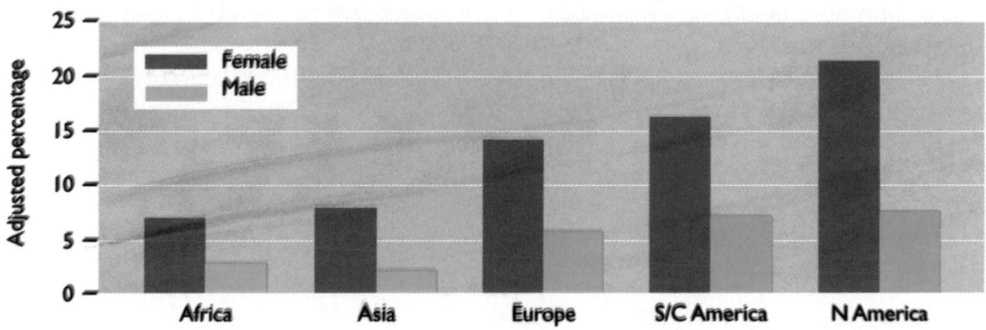


**Figure 3.2** Adjusted prevalence of migraine by geographic area. Adapted with permission from Stewart WF, Lipton RB, Celentano DD, Reed ML. Prevalence of migraine headache in the United States. Relation to age, income, race, and other sociodemographic factors. *JAMA* 1992;267:64–9

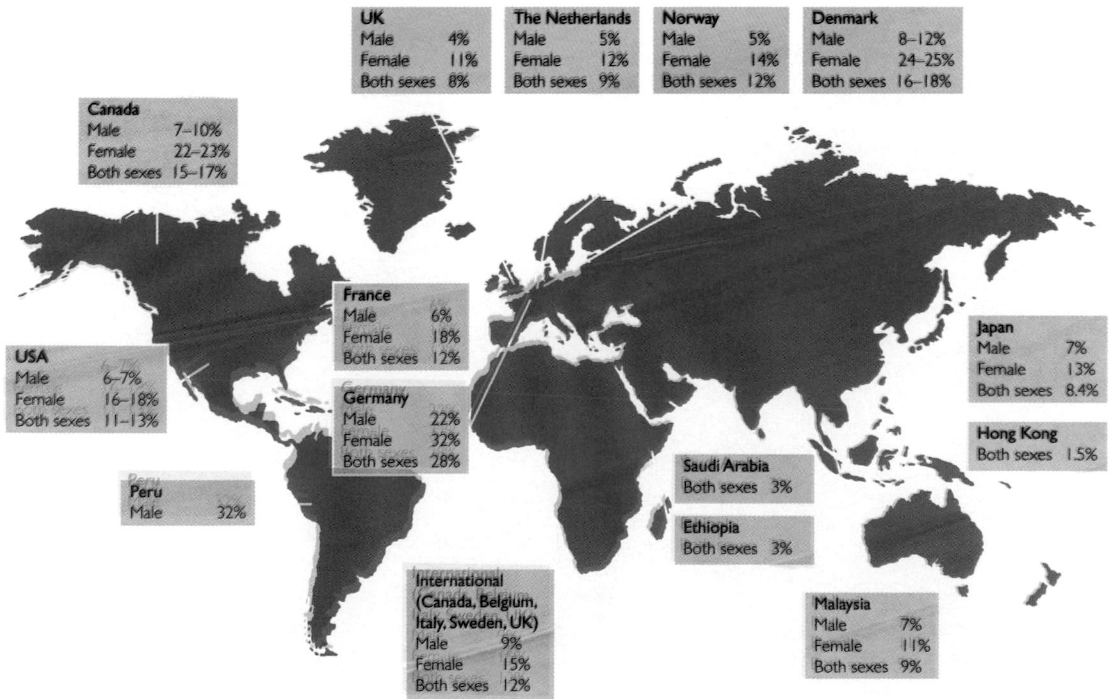


**Figure 3.3** Estimates of migraine prevalence in studies using the diagnostic criteria of the International Headache Society (IHS). Adapted with kind permission of Richard B. Lipton

respectively. In the American Migraine Study, the one-year prevalence of migraine increased with age among women and men, reaching the maximum at ages 35–45 and declining thereafter (Figures 3.5 and 3.6). Migraine prevalence is inversely proportional to income, with the low income groups having the highest prevalence (Figure 3.7). Ethnicity and geographic region also influence migraine prevalence[4]. It is highest in North America and Western Europe, and more prevalent among Caucasians than African- or Asian-Americans. Migraine is influenced by environmental and genetic factors. Migraine with aura has a stronger genetic influence than migraine without aura and is influenced more by environmental factors. Behavioral, emotional and climatologic changes may trigger migraine, modify the vulnerability to migraine or impact on its prevalence.

Evidence suggests that the incidence of migraine may be increasing. Stang *et al.*[7], in a population-based survey of migraine conducted from 1979–1981 in Olmsted County, found that there was a striking increase in the age-adjusted incidence of migraine in those under 45 years of age. Migraine incidence increased by 34% for women and by 100% for men. In this study, the overall age-adjusted incidence was 137 per 100 000 individuals per year for men and 294 per 100 000 individuals per year for women.

In contrast, the American Migraine Study II, a follow-up to the original American Migraine Study, showed that the prevalence of migraine in the United States is 18.2% for women and 6.5% for men. This is essentially unchanged from the original study (prevalence 17.6% and 5.7%, respectively). The

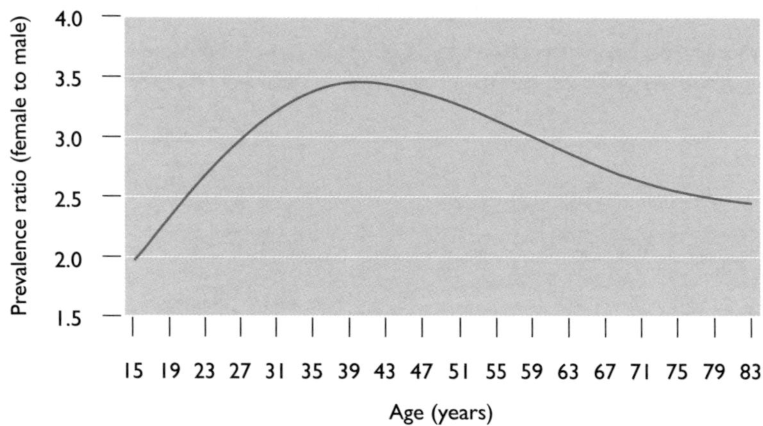


**Figure 3.4** Women are more commonly affected by headache than men. This graph shows the prevalence ratio of migraine headache (females to males) over a lifetime. Adapted with permission from Lipton RB, Stewart WF. Migraine in the United States: a review of epidemiology and health care use. *Neurology* 1993;43(Suppl 3):S6–10

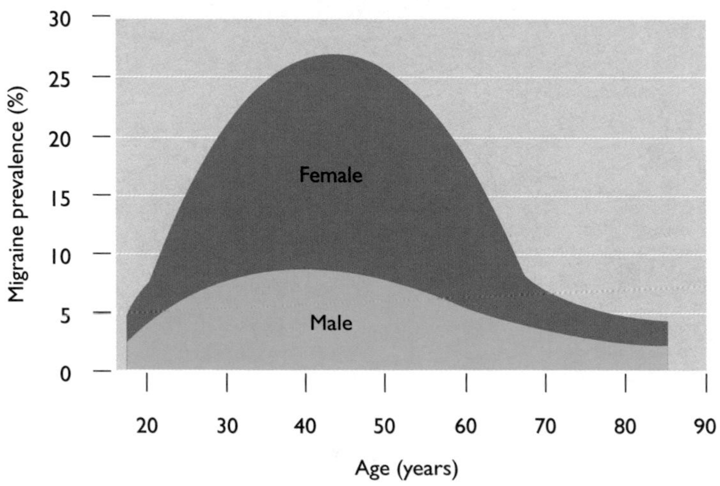


**Figure 3.5** Age-specific prevalence of migraine among women and men in a US study. Adapted with permission from Stewart WF, Lipton RB, Celentano DD, Reed ML. Prevalence of migraine headache in the United States. *JAMA* 1992;267:64–9

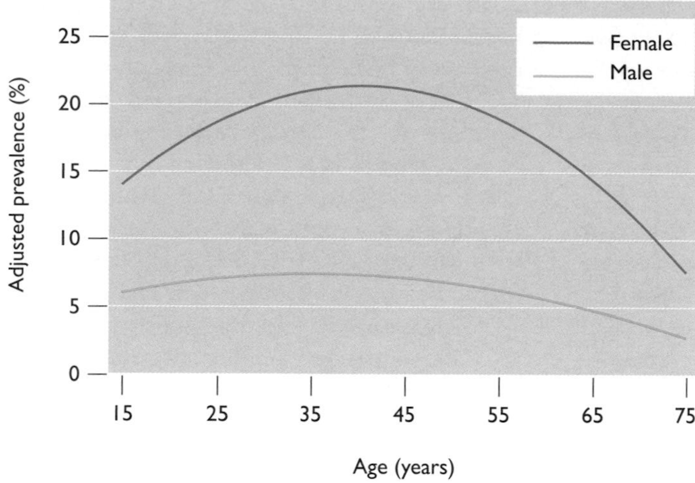


**Figure 3.6** Age- and sex-specific prevalence of migraine based on a meta-analytic summary of 18 population-based studies. Adapted with permission from Scher AI, Stewart WF, Lipton RB. Migraine and headache: A meta-analytic approach. In: Crombie I, ed. *Epidemiology of Pain*. Seattle: IASP Press, 1999:159–70

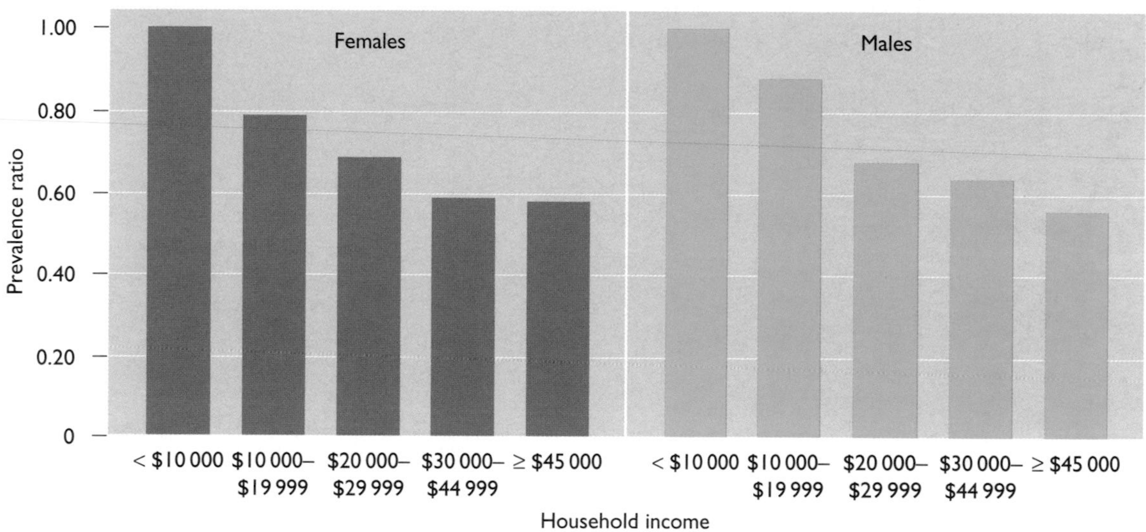


**Figure 3.7** Migraine prevalence is inversely proportional to income, with the low income groups having the highest prevalence. Adapted with permission from Lipton RB, Stewart WF, Celentano DD, Reed ML. Undiagnosed migraine headaches. A comparison of symptom-based and reported physician diagnosis. *Arch Intern Med* 1992;152:1273–8

distribution of disease by sociodemographic factors has remained stable over the last decade, and migraine continues to be more prevalent in Caucasians than in other ethnic groups and in the lower income groups.

## Impact and costs

Migraine is a public health problem of enormous scope that has an impact on both the individual sufferer and on society. Migraine is a lifelong, common disorder that affects people during their most productive years. The individual burden accounts for the impact of attacks on quality of life, and reduction of family, social and recreational activities. The societal burden refers to direct costs, primarily the cost of medical care, and indirect costs, which are due to the impact on work (absenteeism and reduced effectiveness; Figure 3.8). The American

Migraine Study estimates that 23 million US residents have severe migraine headaches. Twenty-five percent of women experience four or more severe attacks a month; 35% experience one to three severe attacks a month; and 40% experience one, or less than one, severe attack a month. Similar frequency patterns were observed for men[4].

In the American Migraine Study, more than 85% of women and more than 82% of men with severe migraine had some headache-related disability. About one-third were severely disabled or needed bed rest (Figure 3.9). As headache pain intensity increases, more migraineurs report disability (Figure 3.10). It is estimated that the typical male migraineur has 3.8 and the typical woman sufferer 5.6 days of bed rest each year, resulting in a total of 112 million bedridden days per year in the US[8]. In addition to the attack-related disability, many migraineurs live in fear, knowing that at any time an attack could disrupt their ability to work, care for their families or meet social obligations. In a prospective diary study, 17% of social and family activities had to be canceled because of headaches[9].

Migraine has an enormous impact on society. In the US, annual lost productivity due to migraine costs 13 billion dollars[3], while direct costs are esti-

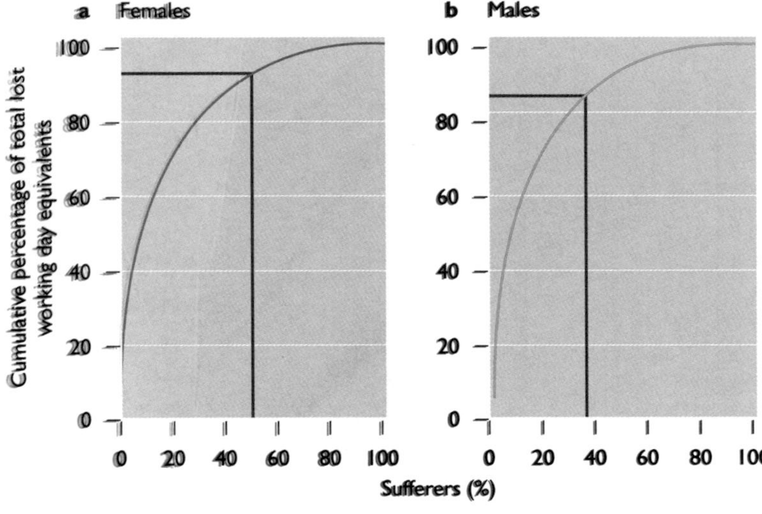


**Figure 3.8** Fifty percent of female migraineurs and almost 40% of male migraineurs accounted for approximately 90% of lost working day equivalents. Adapted with permission from Stewart WF, Lipton RB, Simon D. Work-related disability: Results from the American Migraine Study. *Cephalalgia* 1996;16:231–8

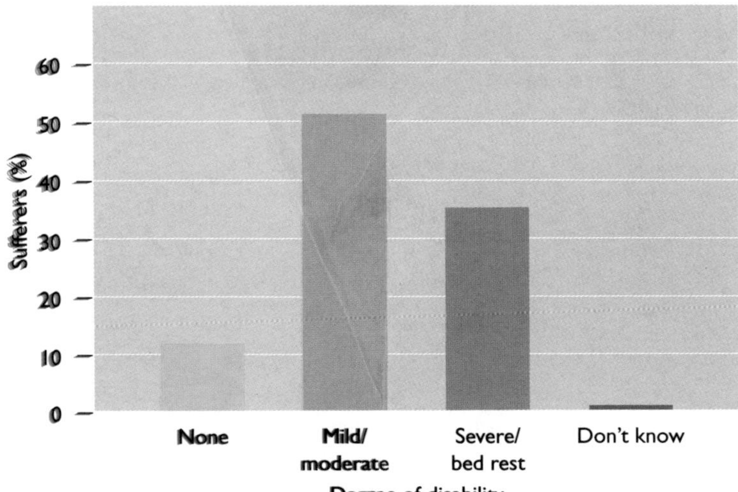


**Figure 3.9** Degree of disability due to migraine in a US study. Adapted with permission from Stewart WF, Lipton RB, Celentano DD, Reed ML. Prevalence of migraine headache in the United States. *JAMA* 1992;267:64–9

mated to be 2.5 billion dollars per year. Migraine's impact on health care utilization is marked as well. The National Ambulatory Medical Care Survey, conducted from 1976–1977, found that 4% of all visits to physicians' offices (over 10 million visits a year) were for headache. Migraine also results in major utilization of emergency rooms and urgent care centers[10].

## Comorbidity

Comorbidity refers to the coexistence of one disorder with another that occurs more commonly than by chance. Stroke, epilepsy, depression, mania, anxiety and panic disorders are comorbid with migraine. Comorbidity has implications for headache diagnosis. Migraine has substantial overlap of symptoms with its comorbid conditions. Both epilepsy and migraine can cause headache and transient alterations of consciousness. Stroke and migraine can both cause transient neurologic signs and headaches. Prodromal migraine symptoms, such as fatigue and irritability, may be part of comorbid depression. Migraine is also a risk factor for a number of comorbid disorders. Comorbidity has important therapeutic implications. Comorbid conditions may impose therapeutic limitations, but therapeutic opportunities may arise as well. For example, antidepressants would be the first option when migraine and depression are concomitant.

In addition to the diagnostic and therapeutic implications, the presence of comorbidity may provide clues to the pathophysiology of migraine. When two conditions occur in the same person, the apparent associations may arise by coincidence, one condition may cause the other or shared environmental or genetic risk factors might account for the co-occurrence of two disorders. For example, head injury is a risk factor for both migraine and epilepsy and may account for part of the relationship between the disorders. Shared genetic risk factors may also account for the association between comorbid disorders. Finally, independent genetic or environmental risk factors may produce a brain state that gives rise to both migraine and a comorbid condition.

## Migraine and stroke

Both migraine and stroke are neurologic disorders that are associated with focal, neurologic signs, alterations in blood flow or headache. The relationship between stroke and migraine could be better understood by the following proposed classification system: (i) coexisting stroke and migraine; (ii) stroke with clinical features of migraine (symptomatic migraine, migraine mimic); (iii) migraine-induced stroke (with and without risk factors); (iv) uncertain[11]. The proportion of strokes attributed to migraine varies from 1–17% in clinical series. Migraine is a risk factor for stroke. The risk of stroke among women under 45 years of age with migraine was three-fold higher than that of controls, and six-fold higher than that of controls for women suffering migraine with aura. Young women with migraine who smoked increased their stroke risk to approximately ten-fold that of controls, and to 14-fold that of controls if they were on oral contraceptives[12].

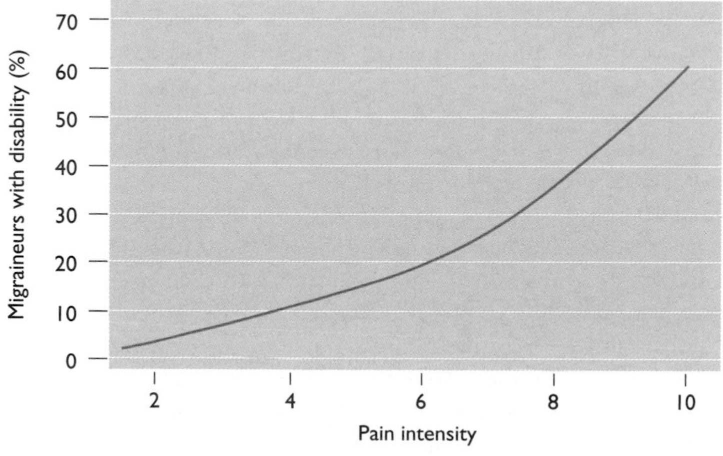


**Figure 3.10** Relationship between disability and headache pain intensity in a group of migraine sufferers. Adapted with permission from Stewart WF, Shechter A, Lipton RB. Migraine heterogeneity. Disability, pain intensity and attack frequency and duration. *Neurology* 1994;44:24–39

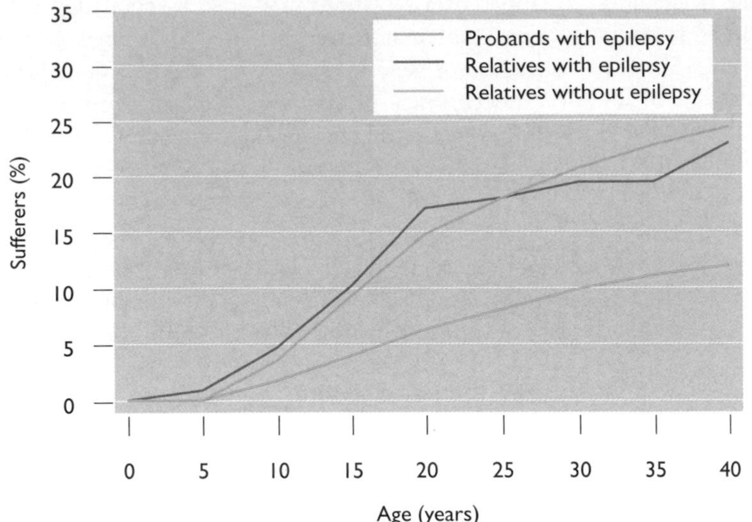


**Figure 3.11** Cumulative incidence of migraine headache, by age, in probands with epilepsy (red), relatives with epilepsy (yellow) and relatives without epilepsy (green). Adapted with permission from Ottman R, Lipton RB. Comorbidity of migraine and epilepsy. *Neurology* 1994;44:2105–10

## Migraine and epilepsy

The prevalence of epilepsy in migraine patients is 5.9%, greatly exceeding the population prevalence of 0.5%. There is a two-fold increase in migraine among both epileptic probands and their relatives[13] (Figure 3.11). The comorbidity of migraine and epilepsy can be explained by a state of neuronal excitability that increases the risk of both disorders. Treatment strategies for patients with comorbid migraine and epilepsy may have limitations, such as drugs that lower seizure threshold (tricyclic antidepressants, neuroleptics), but anticonvulsants (topiramate, divalproex) are drugs of choice for this association.

## Migraine and psychiatric disorders

Several population-based studies have examined the comorbidity of migraine, major depression, panic disorder and other psychiatric disorders. Stewart *et al.*[14] found that 15% of women and 12.8% of men with headache between the ages of 24–29 years had panic disorder. Migraine headache was higher in individuals with a history of panic disorder. The relative risk was 7.0 for men and 3.7 in women.

Merikangas *et al.*[15] found that anxiety and affective disorders were more common in migraineurs. The odds ratio was 2.2 for depression, 2.9 for bipolar spectrum disorders, 2.7 for generalized anxiety disorder, 3.3 for panic disorder, 2.4 for simple phobia and 3.4 for social phobia. Major depression and anxiety disorders were commonly found together. In individuals with all three disorders, the onset of anxiety generally precedes the onset of migraine, whereas the onset of major depression usually follows the onset of migraine.

Breslau *et al.*[16] found that lifetime rates of affective and anxiety disorders were elevated in migraineurs. After adjusting for sex, the odds ratios were 4.5 for major depression, 6.0 for manic episode, 3.2 for any anxiety disorder and 6.6 for panic disorder. Migraine with aura was more strongly associated with the various psychiatric disorders than was migraine without aura.

Personality disorders have been linked to migraine. Brandt *et al.*[17] used the Eysenck Personality Questionnaire (EPQ) in the Washington County Migraine Prevalence Study sample. The EPQ is a well-standardized measure that includes four scales: psychoticism (P), extroversion (E), neuroticism (N) and lie (L). Migraineurs had higher scores than controls on the EPQ N scale, indicating that they were more tense, anxious and depressed than the control group. Women with migraine scored significantly higher than controls on the P scale, indicating that they were more hostile, less interpersonally sensitive and out of step with their peers.

Chronic daily headache, particularly chronic migraine, is highly comorbid with depression, anxiety and insomnia[18]. Fibromyalgia is present in 35% of chronic migraine patients, and it is associated with depression and insomnia[19].

## REFERENCES

1. Rasmussen BK, Jensen R, Schroll M, Olesen J. Epidemiology of headache in a general population – a prevalence study. *J Clin Epidemiol* 1991;44: 1147–57

2. Rasmussen BK, Olesen J. Symptomatic and non-symptomatic headaches in a general population. *Neurology* 1992;42:1225–31

3. Russell MB, Rasmussen BK, Thorvaldsen P, Olesen J. Prevalence and sex-ratio of the subtypes of migraine. *Int J Epidemiol* 1995;24:612–18

4. Stewart WF, Lipton RB, Celentano DD, Reed ML. Prevalence of migraine headache in the United States. *JAMA* 1992;267:64–9

5. Henry P, Michel P, Brochet B, *et al.* A nationwide survey of migraine in France: prevalence and clinical features in adults. GRIM. *Cephalalgia* 1992;12: 229–37

6. Morillo LE, Sanin LC, Takeuchi Y, *et al.* Headache in Latin America: a multination population-based survey. *Neurology* 2001;56:A544 (abstract)

7. Stang PE, Yanagihara PA, Swanson JW, *et al.* Incidence of migraine headache: a population-based study in Olmsted County, Minnesota. *Neurology* 1992; 42:1657–62

8. Hu XH, Markson LE, Lipton RB, *et al.* Burden of migraine in the United States: disability and economic costs. *Arch Intern Med* 1999;159:813–18

9. Edmeads J, Findlay H, Tugwell P, *et al.* Impact of migraine and tension-type headache on life-style, consulting behavior, and medication use: a Canadian population survey. *Can J Neurol Sci* 1993;20:131–7

10. Celentano DD, Stewart WF, Lipton RB, Reed ML. Medication use and disability among migraineurs: a national probability sample. *Headache* 1992;32: 223–8

11. Welch KM. Relationship of stroke and migraine. *Neurology* 1994;44:S33–6

12. Carolei A, Marini C, De Matteis G. History of migraine and risk of cerebral ischaemia in young adults. The Italian National Research Council Study Group on Stroke in the Young. *Lancet* 1996;347: 1503–6

13. Ottman R, Lipton RB. Is the comorbidity of epilepsy and migraine due to a shared genetic susceptibility? *Neurology* 1996;47:918–24

14. Stewart WF, Shechter A, Liberman J. Physician consultation for headache pain and history of panic: results from a population-based study. *Am J Med* 1992;92:35S–40S

15. Merikangas KR, Angst J, Isler H. Migraine and psychopathology. Results of the Zurich cohort study of young adults. *Arch Gen Psychiatry* 1990;47: 849–53

16. Breslau N, Davis GC. Migraine, major depression and panic disorder: a prospective epidemiologic study of young adults. *Cephalalgia* 1992;12:85–9

17. Brandt J, Celentano D, Stewart WF, *et al.* Personality and emotional disorder in a community sample of migraine headache sufferers. *Am J Psychiatry* 1990; 147:303–8

18. Mathew NT. Transformed migraine. *Cephalalgia* 1993;13:78–83

19. Peres MFP, Young WB, Zukerman E, *et al.* Fibromyalgia is common in patients with transformed migraine. *Neurology* 2001;57:1326–8

# 4

# Pathophysiology of headache

Michael L Oshinsky

## ANATOMY OF HEADACHE

The fifth cranial, or trigeminal, nerve arises from the trigeminal ganglion. It transmits somatic sensory information from the head, face and dura to the CNS. The trigeminal nerve has three divisions: ophthalmic, mandibular, and maxillary. Anterior structures of the head and face are innervated by the ophthalmic (first) division. Posterior regions are innervated by the upper cervical nerves. The trigeminal nerve enters the brain stem at the pontine level and terminates in the trigeminal brain stem nuclear complex. The trigeminal brain stem nuclear complex is composed of the principal trigeminal nuclei and spinal trigeminal nuclei (subdivided into the nucleus oralis, the subnuclear interpolaris, and the nucleus caudalis). The brain stem spinal trigeminal nucleus is analogous to the dorsal horn of the spinal chord. The trigeminothalamic tract is analogous to the spinothalamic tract. Second-order neurons from the trigeminal spinal nuclei form the trigeminothalamic tract and project to other midbrain structures, as well as to the thalamus.

## PAIN IN MIGRAINE

Migraine is a primary brain disorder, a form of neurovascular headache in which neural events result in dilation of blood vessels and nociceptive afferent activation. Three components seem to be involved in migraine pain: (1) the cranial blood vessels, (2) the trigeminal innervation of the vessels, and (3) the reflex connections of the trigeminal system and the cranial parasympathetic system (Figure 4.1). The key pathway for headache pain is trigeminovascular input from the meningeal vessels. Brain imaging studies suggest that important modulation of the trigeminovascular nociceptive input stems from the dorsal raphe nucleus (Figure 4.2), locus coeruleus, and nucleus raphe magnus.

## PERIPHERAL MECHANISMS/NOCICEPTOR ACTIVATION

During a migraine attack, an inflammatory process (neurogenic inflammation) occurs at the site of the nerve terminal[1]. Trigeminal afferent activation is accompanied by the release of vasoactive neuropeptides, including calcitonin gene-related peptide (CGRP), substance P (SP), and neurokinin A, from the nerve terminals. These mediators produce mast cell activation, sensitization of the nerve terminals, and extravasation of fluid into the perivascular space around the dural blood vessels (Figure 4.3). Intense neuronal stimulation causes induction of *c-fos* (an immediate early gene product) in the trigeminal nucleus caudalis (TNC) of the brainstem. Substance P and CGRP further amplify the trigeminal terminal sensitivity by stimulating the release of bradykinin and other inflammatory mediators from mast cells. Prostaglandins and nitric oxide (a diffusible gas that acts as a neurotransmitter) are both endogenous mediators that can be produced locally and can sensitize nociceptors. Cortical spreading depression (the cause of the migraine aura) can also activate nociceptors of the trigeminal system (Figures 4.4–4.11). Although the brain itself is largely insensate, pain can be generated by large cranial vessels and the dura mater. The involvement of the ophthalmic division of the trigeminal nerve and its overlap of structures

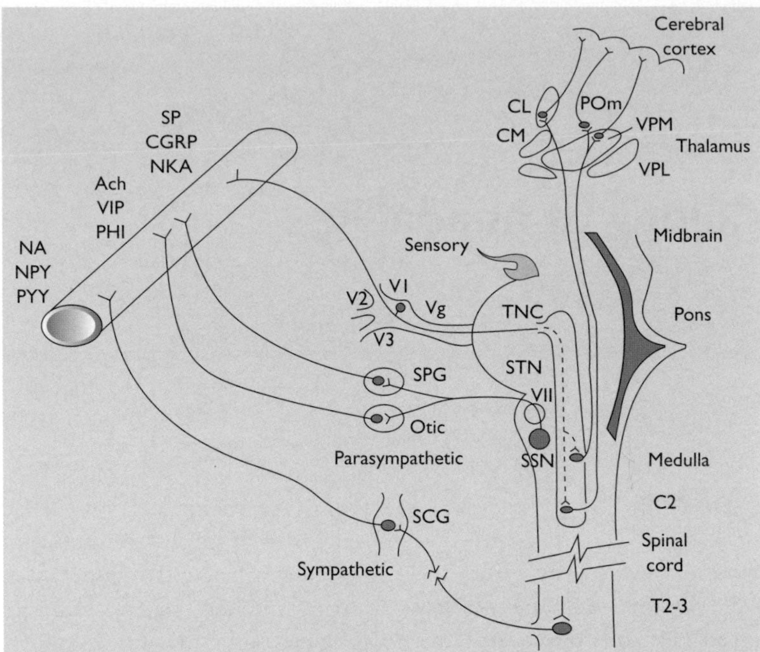


**Figure 4.1** Brainstem nuclei and their transmitters. Ach, acetylcholine; C2, second cervical segment of the spinal cord; CGRP, calcitonin gene-related peptide; CL, centrolateral nucleus of thalamus; CM, centromedial nucleus of thalamus; NA, noradrenaline; NKA, neurokinin A; NPY, neuropeptide Y; Otic, otic ganglion; PHI, peptide histidine isoleucine (methionine in man); POm, medial nucleus of the posterior complex; PYY, peptide YY; SCG, superior cervical ganglion; SP, substance P; SPG, sphenopalatine ganglion; SSN, superior salivatory nucleus; STN, spinal trigeminal nucleus; T2-3, second and third thoracic segments of the spinal cord; TNC, trigeminal nucleus caudalis; VII, seventh cranial nerve (parasympathetic outflow); VIP, vasoactive intestinal polypeptide; VPL, ventroposterolateral nucleus of thalamus; VPM, ventroposteromedial nucleus of thalamus; Vg, trigeminal ganglion; VI-3, first, second and third divisions of the trigeminal nerve. Reproduced with permission from Goadsby PJ, Zagami AS, Lambert GA. Neural processing of craniovascular pain: a synthesis of the central structures involved in migraine. *Headache* 1991;31:365–71

innervated by branches of C2 nerve roots explain the typical distribution of migraine pain over the frontal and temporal regions and the referral of pain to the parietal, occipital, and high cervical regions.

## SENSITIZATION IN MIGRAINE

Clinicians have observed that, during migraine attacks, patients complain of increased pain with stimuli that would ordinarily be non-nociceptive[2]. These stimuli include hair brushing, wearing a hat, and resting the head on a pillow. This phenomenon of pain induction by nonpainful stimuli is referred to as allodynia. Burstein et al. explored the development of allodynia in patients with migraine. He measured pain thresholds for hot, cold, and pressure stimuli, both within the region of spontaneous pain and outside it[3]. He found that as one attack progressed in a selected group of migraine sufferers, cutaneous allodynia developed in the region of pain and then outside it at extracephalic locations. He found that 33 of 42 patients (79%) developed allodynia.

Sensitizations of nociceptors or secondary sensory neurons in the TNC are the physiological cause of clinical symptoms of allodynia. The afferent or the central neurons processing the sensory information may have an increased spontaneous discharge rate or increased responsiveness to both painful and non-painful stimuli. The receptor fields of these neurons can expand, resulting in pain being felt over a greater part of the dermatome. This results in hyperalgesia (increased sensitivity to pain) and cutaneous allodynia (pain perceived in response to non-painful stimuli). Peripheral sensitization produces localized increased pain sensitivity.

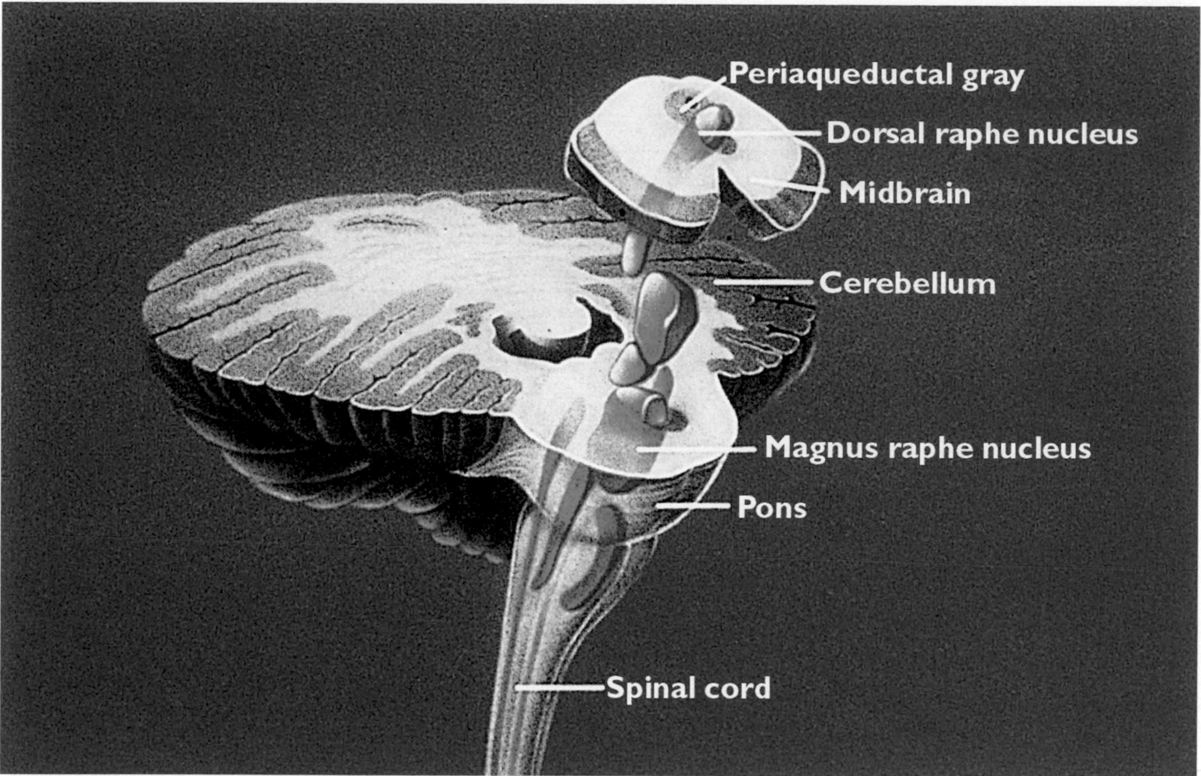


**Figure 4.2** Brainstem nuclei thought to be involved in migraine generation include the periaqueductal gray matter and dorsal raphe nucleus

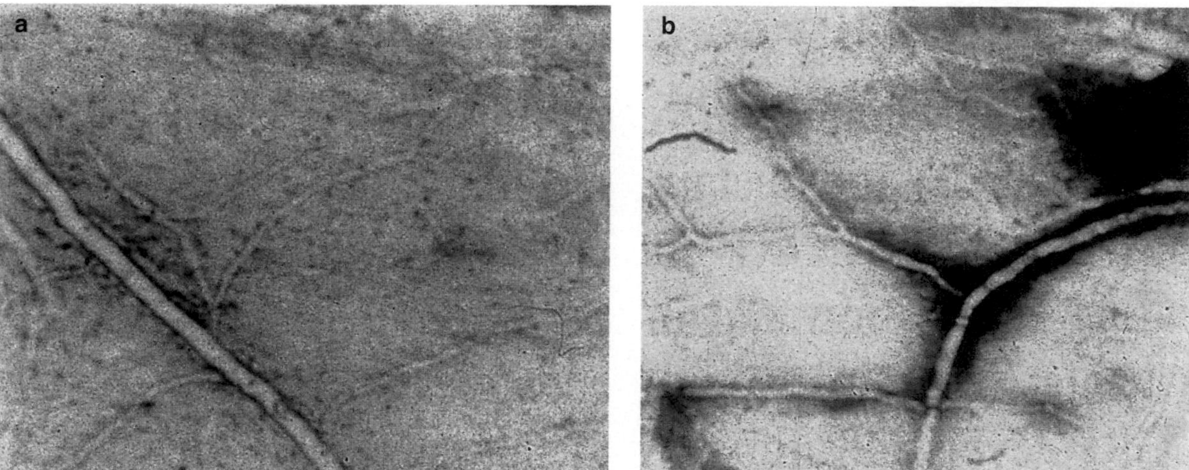


**Figure 4.3** Trigeminal stimulation in the rat produces plasma protein extravasation. 5-Hydroxytryptamine receptor agonists for the abortive treatment of vascular headaches block this effect. (a) control; (b) stimulated. Reproduced from Buzzi MG, Dimitriadou V, Theoharides TC, Moskowitz MA. 5-Hydroxytryptamine receptor agonists for the abortive treatment of vascular headaches block mast cell, endothelial and platelet activation within the rat dura mater after trigeminal stimulation. *Brain Res* 1992;583:137–49, with permission of Elsevier Science

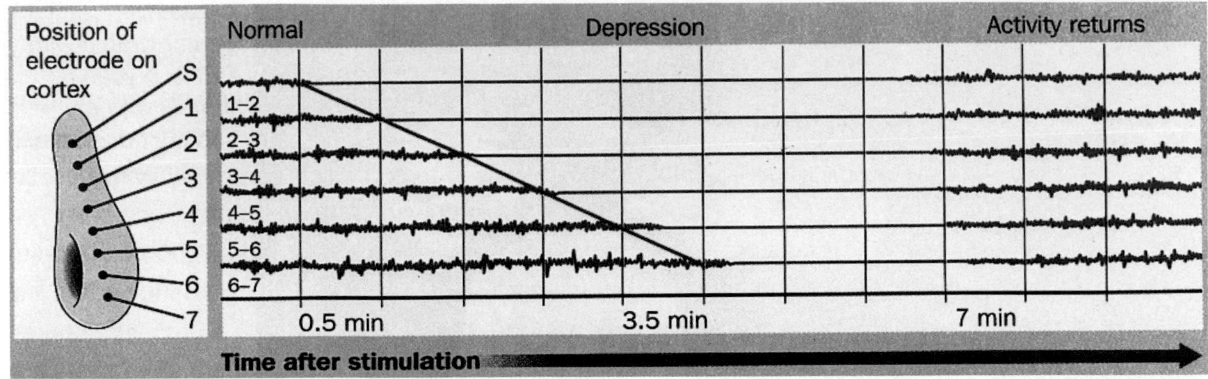


**Figure 4.4** Leao found that noxious stimulation of the exposed cortex of a rabbit produced a spreading decrease in electrical activity that moved at a rate of 2–3 mm/min. Reading from the rabbit cortex illustrating spreading depression of EEG activity. Reproduced with permission from Leao AAP. Spreading depression of activity in cerebral cortex. *J Neurophysiol* 1944;7:359–90

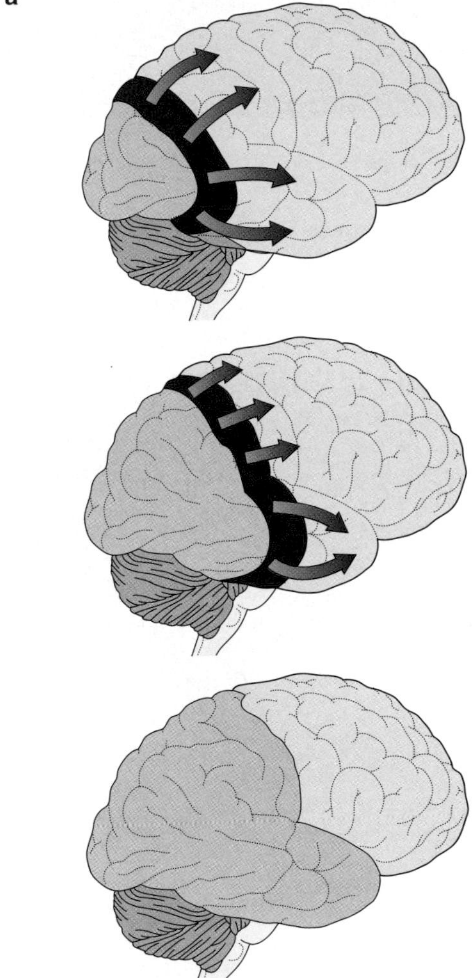


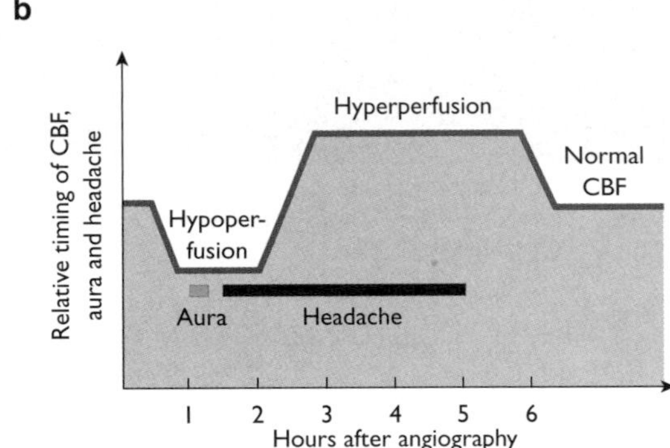


**Figure 4.5** Line drawing (panel a) of the spreading oligemia observed with studies of cerebral blood flow (CBF) during aura after Lauritzen. Adapted with permission from Lauritzen M. Cortical spreading depression as a putative migraine mechanism. *Trends Neurosci* 1987;10:8–13, with permission from Elsevier Science. Panel b illustrates the variable time course and relationship of the changes in cerebral blood flow and the symptomatology of migraine. Adapted with permission from Olesen J, Friberg L, Skyhoj-Olesen T, *et al*. Timing and topography of cerebral blood flow, aura and headache during migraine attacks. *Ann Neurol* 1990;28:791–8

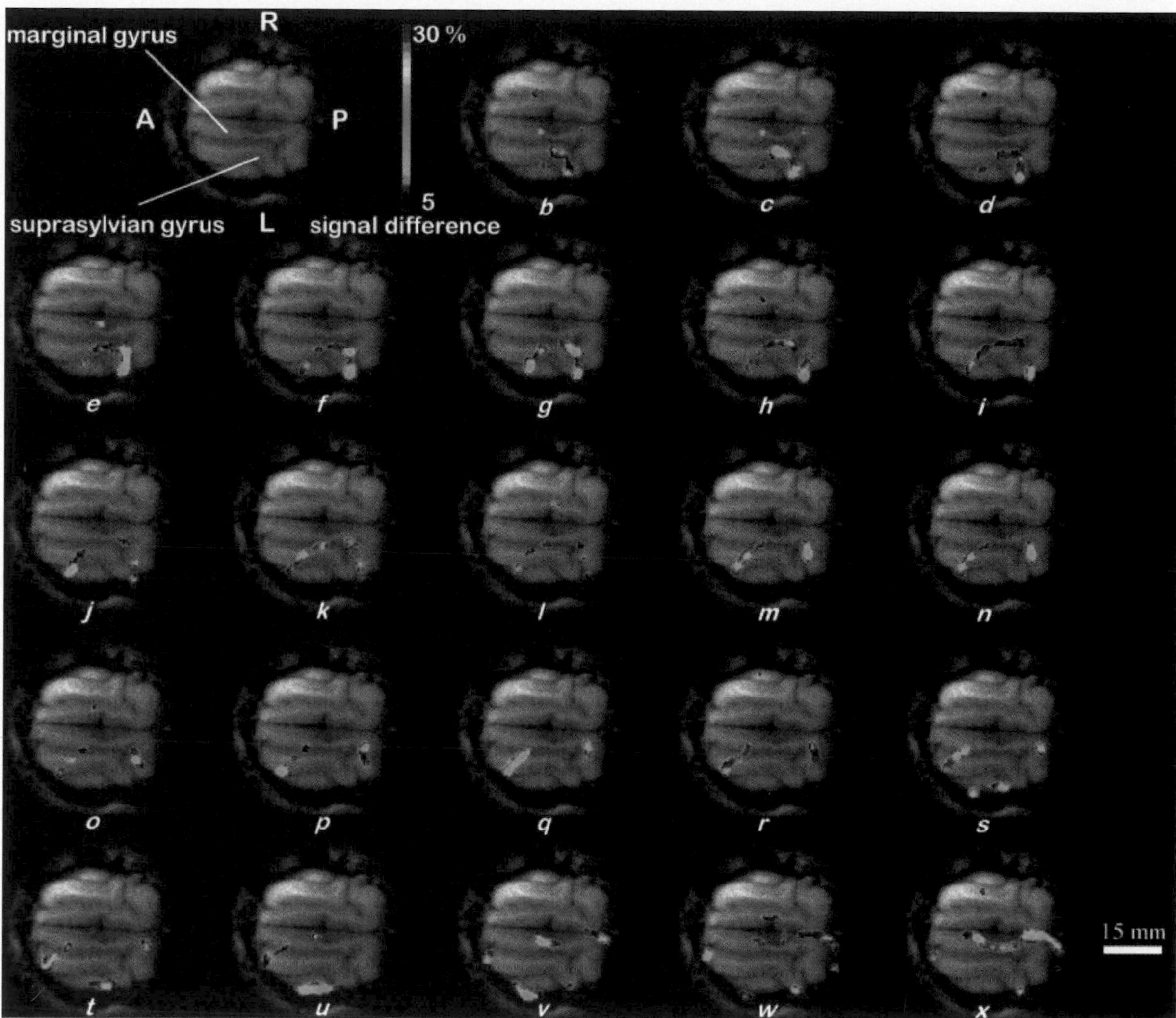


**Figure 4.6** Propagation of cortical spreading depression (CSD) across the surface of the cat brain *in vivo*. Top left, control, horizontal, gradient-echo anatomic image depicting the suprasylvian and marginal gyri. Remaining images (b-x): coloured overlays, shown at 10 s intervals starting about 50 s after KCl application, represent elliptical regions of reduced diffusion travelling away from the KCl application site with a velocity of 3.2 ± 0.1 mm/min (mean ± SEM of 5 measurements). Over the first eleven frames (b-i) the wave travels both rostrally and caudally along the suprasylvian gyrus; when it reaches the caudal junction of the two gyri (m-s), it appears to pass into the marginal gyrus (t-x); likewise, rostrally, the wave passes first (r-x) into the ectosylvian gyrus where it dissipates (v–x) and then into the marginal gyrus (t–x). Waves were never detected in the contralateral hemisphere. A, anterior; P, posterior; R, right; L, left; overlays were obtained by subtracting a baseline image from the high-b images obtained in the DWEP sequence and transforming the signal difference into a percentage change (blue 5%, red 30%). Scale bar, 15 mm. This image represents the first reported detection of CSD with magnetic resonance imaging (MRI) in a species which shares with man a complex, gyrencephalic brain structure. Reproduced with permission from James MF, Smith MI, Bockhorst KH, *et al*. Cortical spreading depression in the gyrencephalic feline brain studied by magnetic resonance imaging. *J Physiol* 1999;519:415–25

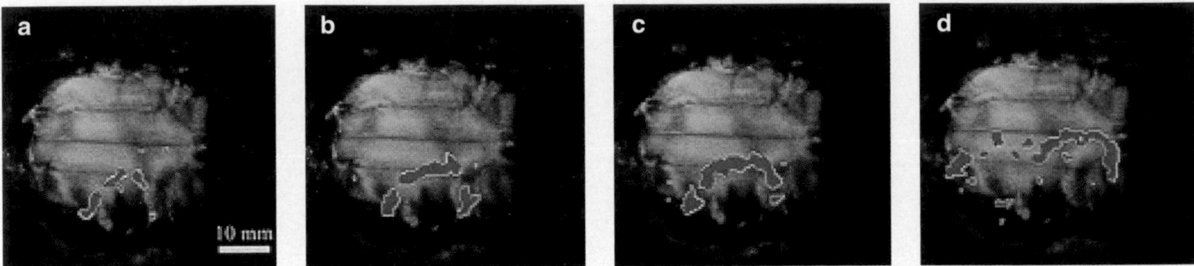


**Figure 4.7** Spreading depression: A model of migraine. Colored overlays of changes in blood oxygenation in an experimental model of cortical spreading depression. Overlays a–d represent the points 0.5, 1.0, 1.4 and 5.1 min post-induction. Reproduced with permission from James MF, Smith MI, Bockhorst KH, *et al*. Cortical spreading depression in the gyrencephalic feline brain studied by magnetic resonance imaging. *J Physiol* 1999;519:415–25

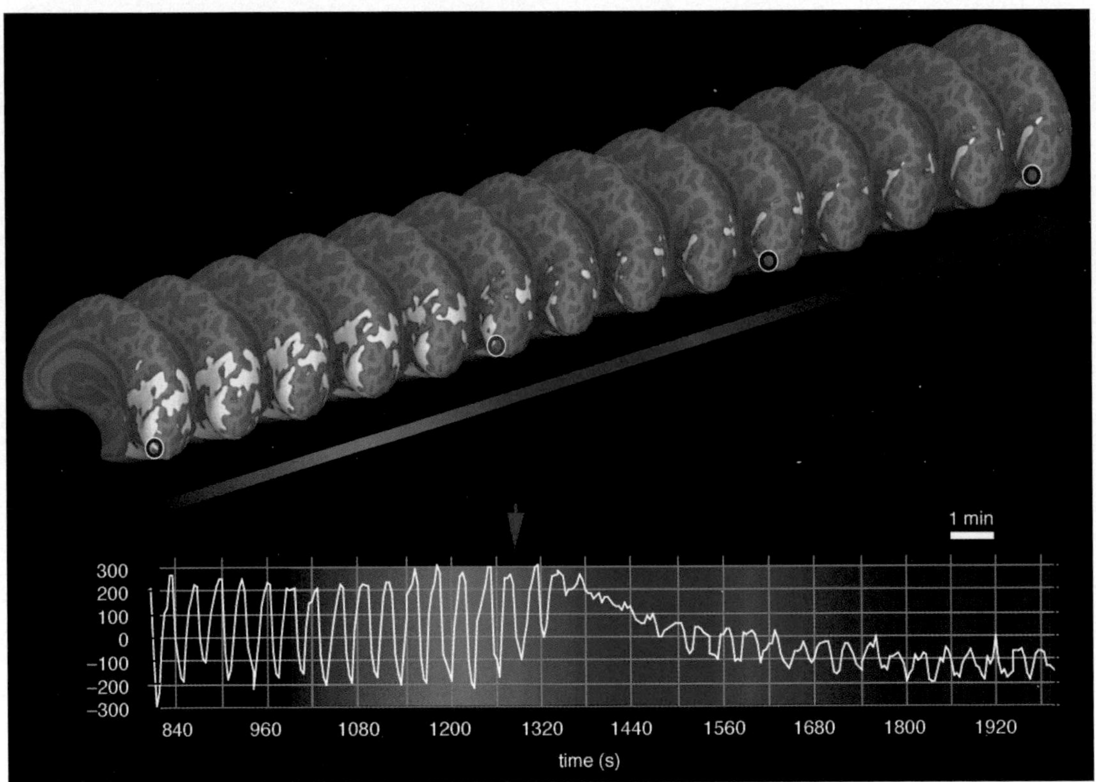


**Figure 4.8** Blood oxygenation level-dependent (BOLD) changes during an exercise-triggered migraine visual aura. Time-dependent BOLD activity changes from a single region of interest in the primary visual cortex (VI), aquired before and during episodes of induced visual aura. The upper panel shows a series of anatomic images, including BOLD activity on 'inflated' cortical hemispheres showing the medial bank (similar to a conventional mid-sagittal view). Images were sampled at 32 s intervals, showing the same region of interest (circle) in VI. The lower panel shows the MR signal perturbation over time from the circled region of interest. Variations in time are color-coded (deep red to magenta) and the four-colored circles match corresponding times within the VI region of interest. Prior to the onset of the aura, the BOLD response to visual stimulation shows a normal, oscillating activation pattern. Following the onset of aura (red arrow), the BOLD response shows a marked increase in mean level and a marked suppression to light modulation followed by a partial recovery of the response to light modulation at a decreased mean level. Reproduced with kind permission of Margarita Sanchez del Rio

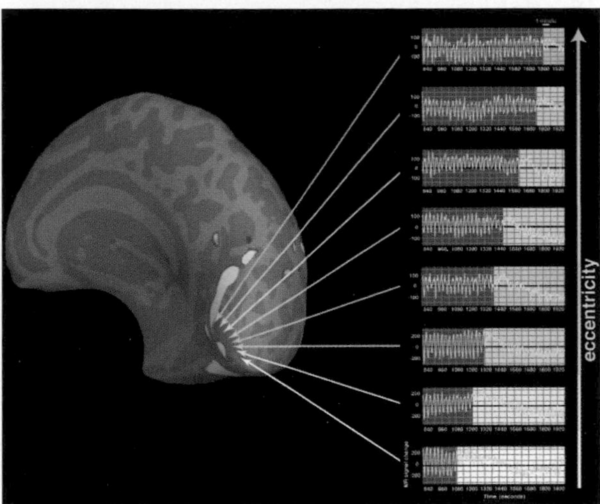


**Figure 4.9** Spreading suppression of cortical activation during migraine visual aura. Data from the same patient as in Figure 4.5. The posterior medial aspect of the occipital lobe is shown in an 'inflated cortex' format. The cortical sulci and gyri appear in darker and lighter gray respectively, on a computationally inflated surface. MR signal changes over time are shown on the right. Each time course was recorded from one in a sequence of voxels which were sampled along the calcarine sulcus in V1, from the posterior pole to the more anterior location, as indicated by the arrow. A similar BOLD response was found within all the extrastriate areas, differing only in the time of onset of the MR perturbation. The MR perturbations developed earlier in the foveal representation, compared to the more eccentric representation of the retinotropic visual cortex. This was consistent with the progression of the aura from central to peripheral eccentricities in the corresponding visual field. Reproduced with kind permission of Margarita Sanchez del Rio

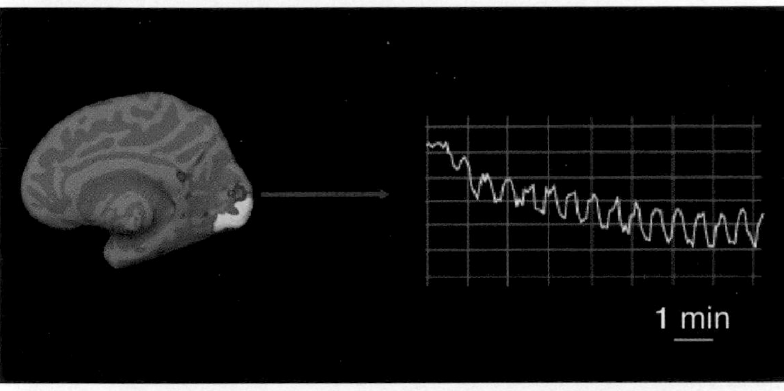


**Figure 4.10** BOLD changes during spontaneous migraine visual aura. Data from a spontaneous attack captured approximately 18 min after the onset of the visual symptoms affecting the right hemifield. The data represent the time course in the left visual area V1, at an eccentricity of approximately 20° of visual angle. BOLD signal changes resemble the changes observed at a similar time point in Figure 4.5. Reproduced with kind permission of Margarita Sanchez del Rio

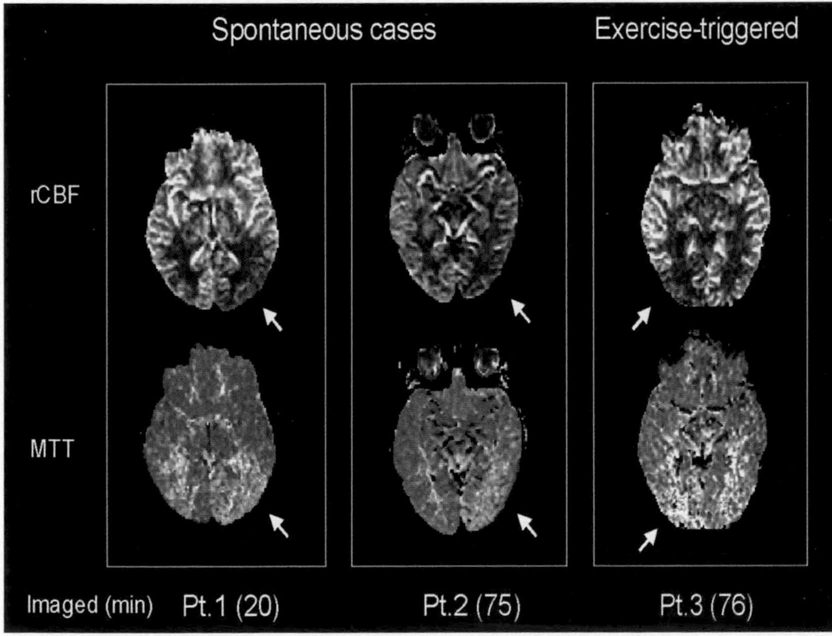


**Figure 4.11** Perfusion weighted imaging (PWI) during migraine with aura attacks. PWI maps obtained at different time points during migraine with aura attacks during the presence of the stereotypical visual aura (patient I, approximately 20 min after onset of visual symptoms) and after resolution of the aura and into the headache phase (patients 2 and 3). In all cases a perfusion defect (decreased rCBF and rCBV, the latter not shown, and increased MTT) was observed in the occipital cortex contralateral to the visual field defect. rCBF, reduced cerebral blood flow; rCBV, regional cerebral blood volume; MTT, mean transit time. Reproduced with kind permission of Margarita Sanchez del Rio

Central sensitization, in contrast, refers to the activity-dependent increase in excitability of nociceptive neurons in the CNS that may outlast afferent input. Since most input received by dorsal horn neurons is sub-threshold, (i.e., the synaptic strength is too weak to evoke an action potential output), after sensitization this normally subthreshold input begins to activate dorsal horn neurons as a result of molecular changes in the pre- and postsynaptic neurons. Central sensitization is characterized by reductions in threshold and increases in the responsiveness of dorsal horn neurons, as well as by enlargement of their receptive fields.

Sensitization results from the activation of multiple intracellular signaling pathways in dorsal horn neurons by the neurotransmitter (glutamate) and the neuromodulators (SP, brain-derived neurotrophic factor, and CGRP)[4]. Cutaneous allodynic pain is referred to the periphery, but it arises from within the central nervous system. Clinically, central sensitization contributes to pain hypersensitivity in the skin and muscle. This can explain the intracranial hypersensitivity (i.e., the worsening pain during coughing, bending over, or any head movement) and the throbbing pain of migraine.

## PAIN MODULATION

The nervous system contains networks that modulate nociceptive transmission[5]. The trigeminal brain stem nuclear complex receives monoaminergic, enkephalinergic, and peptidergic projections from regions known to be important in modulation of the nociceptive systems. A descending inhibitory neuronal network extends from the frontal cortex and hypothalamus through the periaqueductal gray to the rostral ventromedial medulla and the medullary and spinal dorsal horn. The rostral ventromedial medulla includes the raphe nuclei and the adjacent reticular formation and projects to the outer laminae of the spinal and medullary dorsal horn. Electrical stimulation or injection of opioids into the periaqueductal gray or rostral ventromedial medulla inhibits neuron activity in the dorsal horn. The periaqueductal gray receives projections from the insular cortex and the amygdala.

These nuclei are believed to modulate the activity of the TNC and dorsal horn neurons. In the rostral ventromedial medulla and periaqueductal gray, three classes of neurons have been identified. ‘Off-cells’ pause immediately before the nociceptive

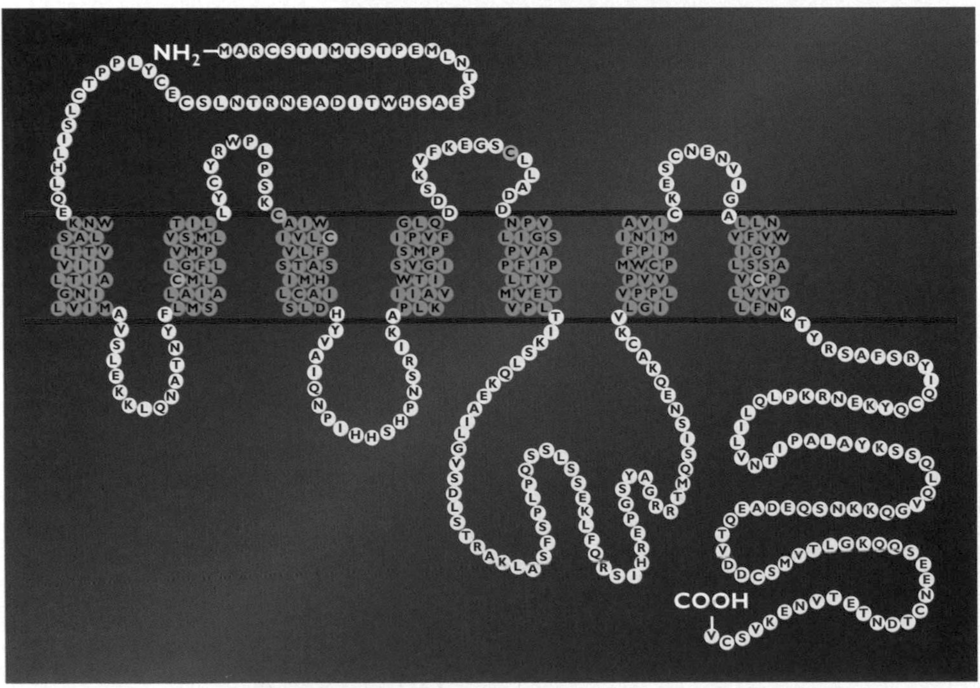


**Figure 4.12** Schematic representation of the primary sequence of the 5-$HT_2$ receptor. Reproduced from Hartig PR. Molecular biology of 5-HT receptor. *Trends Pharmacol Sci* 1989;10:64–9, with permission of Elsevier Science

reflex, whereas 'on-cells' are activated[6,7]. Neutral cells show no consistent changes in activation. Increased on-cell activity in the brain stem's pain modulation system enhances the response to both painful and nonpainful stimuli. Headache may be caused, in part, by enhanced neuronal activity in the nucleus caudalis as a result of enhanced on-cell or decreased off-cell activity. Other conditioned stimuli associated with pain and stress also can turn on the pain system and may account, in part, for the association between pain and stress.

Positron emission tomography performed during a primary headache, such as migraine and cluster headache, has demonstrated activations in brain areas associated with pain, such as the cingulate cortex, insulae, frontal cortex, thalamus, basal ganglia, and cerebellum. These areas are similarly activated when head pain is induced by injecting capsaicin into the forehead of volunteers. In addition to the generic pain areas activated by the capsaicin injections, specific brainstem areas, such as the dorsal pons, are activated in episodic migraine[8,9].

## SUMMARY

Although clinical and basic science research has revealed many pieces of the puzzle of migraine pathophysiology, the full picture is still elusive. For example, we know that environmental and behavior triggers, such as lack of sleep, too much sleep, fasting, thirst etc., can initiate a migraine attack; however, the mechanism by which these triggers initiate the migraine is not clear[10]. Many of these triggers are related to hypothalamic function. Most of the basic science research in migraine has focused on the pain phase of the disorder and has ignored the prodrome and resolution phases. Understanding these aspects of migraine and recognizing that it is more than just a pain disorder is going to be critical to fully elucidate its pathophysiology.

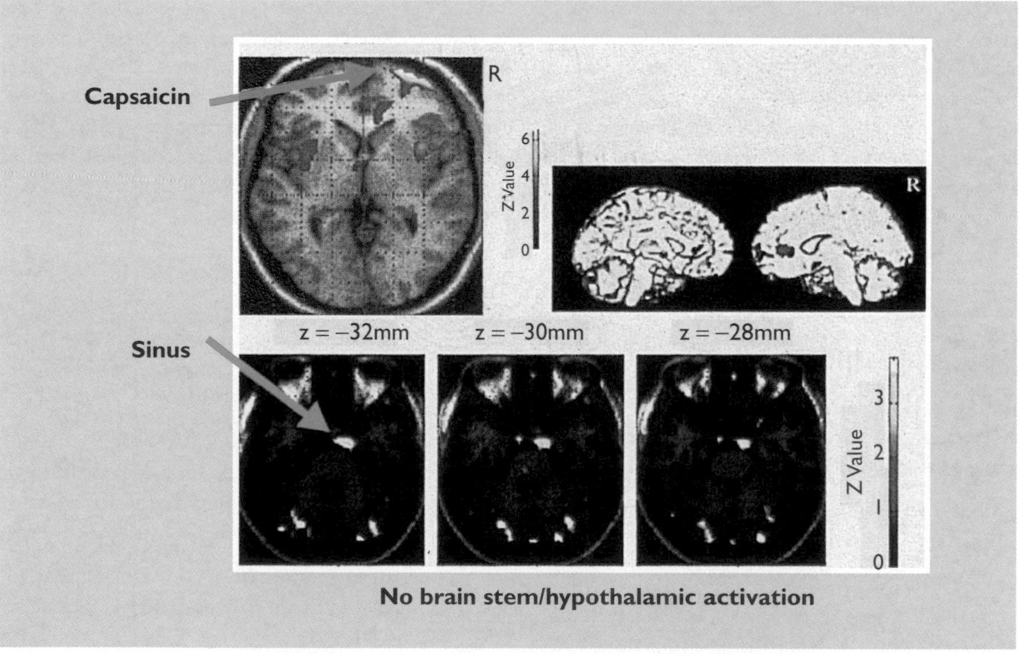


**Figure 4.13** An experimental pain study was conducted in healthy volunteers to further test whether brain stem neuronal activation during migraine is specific to the generation of migraine symptoms. In this study, capsaicin was injected subcutaneously into the right forehead to evoke a painful burning sensation in the first division of the trigeminal nerve. The monoaminergic brain stem regions (raphe nucleus and the locus coeruleus) and the periaqueductal gray were not activated in the acute pain state compared to the pain-free state. Thus, brain stem activation during a migraine attack is probably not a generalized response to head pain but instead represents sites in the nervous system that may give rise to migraine symptomatology. Adapted with permission from May A, Kaube H, Buchel C, *et al.* Experimental cranial pain elicited by capsaicin: a PET study. *Pain* 1998;74:61–6

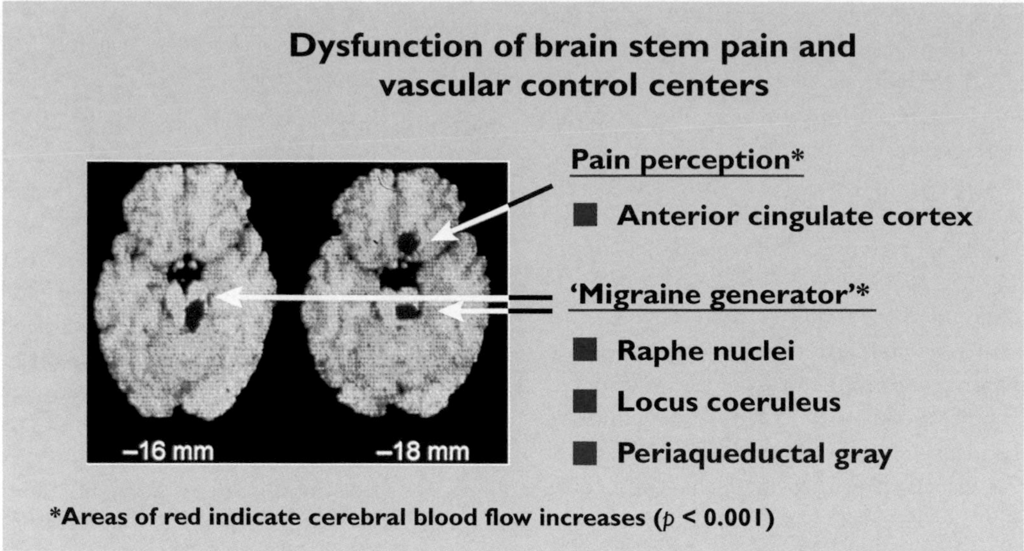


**Figure 4.14** The development of migraine, e.g. episodes in patients undergoing surgery to implant electrodes in the periaqueductal gray and raphe nuclei for the treatment of chronic pain, generated the hypothesis that CNS dysfunction early in the migraine attack could provoke changes in these brain stem nuclei. Weiller *et al.* used positron emission tomography (PET) to examine the changes in regional cerebral blood flow, an index of neuronal activity, during spontaneous migraine attacks. The left panel above is a PET scan from an individual during a migraine attack treated acutely with sumatriptan. The scan depicts neuronal activity in a section through the brain stem. The authors of this study reported that monoaminergic brain stem regions (raphe nucleus comprising serotonergic neurons and the locus coeruleus comprising noradrenergic neurons) and the periaqueductal gray are selectively activated during a migraine attack. When this patient used subcutaneous sumatriptan to acutely relieve his headache pain, the brain stem centers continued to appear active on the follow-up PET scans. By contrast, the anterior cingulate cortex, a region thought to be involved in processing affective components of pain, was also activated during spontaneous migraine attacks, and this activation was reduced concomitantly with headache pain relief after administration of sumatriptan. Taken together, these observations suggest that the raphe nucleus, locus coeruleus and the periaqueductal gray are regions that may be involved in the generation of headache pain and associated symptoms during a migraine attack. Adapted with permission from Weiller C, May A, Limmroth V, *et al.* Brain stem activation in spontaneous human migraine attacks. *Nat Med* 1995;1:658–60

## REFERENCES


1. Reuter U, Bolay H, Jansen-Olesen I, *et al.* Delayed inflammation in rat meninges: implications for migraine pathophysiology. *Brain* 2001;124:2490–2502
2. Drummond PD, Lance JW. Clinical diagnosis and computer analysis of headache symptoms. *J Neurol Neurosurg Psychiatry* 1984;47:128–33
3. Burstein R, Cutrer MF, Yarnitsky D. The development of cutaneous allodynia during a migraine attack clinical evidence for the sequential recruitment of spinal and supraspinal nociceptive neurons in migraine. *Brain* 2000;123:1703–9
4. Millan MJ. The induction of pain: an integrative review. Prog Neurobiol 1999;57:1–164
5. Millan MJ. Descending control of pain. *Progr Neurobiol* 2002;66:355–474
6. Fields HL, Basbaum AI. Central nervous system mechanisms of pain modulation. In: *The Textbook of Pain*. 4th edn. 1999:309
7. Fields HL, Malick A, Burstein R. Dorsal horn projection targets of ON and OFF cells in the rostral ventromedial medulla. *J Neurophysiol* 1995;74:1742–59
8. Goadsby PJ. Neurovascular headache and a midbrain vascular malformation: evidence for a role of the brainstem in chronic migraine. *Cephalalgia* 2002;22:107–11
9. Goadsby PJ. Neuroimaging in headache. *Microsc Res Tech* 2001;53:179–87
10. Malick A, Jakubowski M, Elmquist JK, *et al.* A neurohistochemical blueprint for pain-induced loss of appetite. *Proc Natl Acad Sci USA* 2001;98:9930–5

# 5
# Migraine

Mario F P Peres

Migraine is a common primary episodic headache disorder. In the United States, more than 17% of women and 6% of men had at least one migraine attack in the last year. Although the term migraine derives from the Greek word 'hemicrania' which means half of the head, it is not always a strictly unilateral headache; it can be bilateral and it is characterized by various combinations of neurologic, gastrointestinal, and autonomic symptoms.

There are many migraine subtypes including migraine without aura, migraine with aura, basilar migraine, familial hemiplegic migraine, status migrainous, and chronic (previously transformed) migraine.

According to the International Headache Society (IHS) classification and diagnostic criteria for primary headaches, certain clinical features must be present and organic disease must be excluded for headaches to qualify as migraine.

To diagnose migraine without aura, five attacks are needed, each lasting 4–72 h and having two of the following four characteristics: unilateral location, pulsating quality, moderate-to-severe intensity, and aggravation by routine physical activity. In addition, the attacks must have at least one of the following: nausea (and/or vomiting) or photophobia and phonophobia.

Four phases of migraine (prodrome, aura, headache and postdrome) are recognized and may occur alone or in combination with any other phase. The prodrome consists of premonitory phenomena generally occurring hours to days before the headache and include mental and mood changes (depression, anger, euphoria), stiff neck, fatigue, yawning, food cravings, fluid retention and increase in urination.

The aura is composed of focal neurologic symptoms that usually precede the headache, lasting in general less than 60 min. Visual symptoms are the most common, such as zigzag or scintillating figures (fortification spectrum), scotomata, distortions is shape and size. Motor, sensory or brainstem disturbances can also occur.

The headache phase is typically characterized by unilateral pain, throbbing, moderate to marked in severity, and aggravated by physical activity. The pain of migraine is invariably accompanied by other features. Nausea occurs in almost 90% of patients, while vomiting occurs in about one-third of migraineurs. Many patients experience sensory hyperexcitability manifested by photophobia, phonophobia, and osmophobia, and seek a dark, quiet room. Other systemic symptoms, including anorexia, blurry vision, diarrhea, abdominal cramps, polyuria, pallor of the face, stiffness and tenderness of the neck, and sweating, may be noted during the headache phase. Impairment of concentration is common; less often there is memory impairment. Depression, fatigue, anxiety, nervousness, and irritability are common. Lightheadedness, rather than true vertigo, and a feeling of faintness may occur.

In the postdrome phase, the pain wanes. Following the headache, the patient may feel tired, washed out, irritable, and listless and may have impaired concentration, scalp tenderness, or mood changes. Some people feel unusually refreshed or euphoric after an attack, while others note depression and malaise.

Migraine comorbidity is a very important issue. Migraine is comorbid with several disorders including stroke and epilepsy. Chronic migraine is particularly more related to psychiatric comorbidity (anxiety, depression), sleep disorders, fibromyalgia, and fatigue.

A number of mechanisms and theories have been proposed to explain the causes of migraine. The strong familial association and the early onset of the disorder suggest that there is an important genetic component and migraine has been considered to be a chanellopathy.

The pain distribution suggests involvement of the trigeminal nerve, trigeminal activation resulting in the release of neuropeptides, producing neurogenic inflammation with increased vascular permeability, and dilation of blood vessel. This is the trigeminal vascular model proposed by Moskowitz.

Muscle contraction and tenderness are another important component in migraine patients. Neurotransmitters including serotonin, dopamine, norepinephrine, glutamate, nitric oxide, GABA, and other substances such as magnesium and melatonin have been also considered in migraine pathophysiology. The concept of central sensitization has been recently recognized as an important mechanism in migraine. A mithocondrial dysfunction has also been proposed as one of the migraine etiologies.

The goals of migraine treatment are to relieve or prevent the pain and associated symptoms of migraine and to optimize the patient's ability to function normally. To achieve these goals patients must learn to identify and avoid headache triggers. Pharmacologic treatment of migraine may be acute (abortive, symptomatic) or preventive (prophylactic). Patients experiencing frequent severe headaches often require both approaches. The choice of treatment should be guided by the presence of comorbid conditions. A concurrent illness should be treated with a single agent when possible and agents that might aggravate a comorbid illness should be avoided. Patients' preferences should also be considered Biofeedback, relaxation techniques, and other behavioral interventions can also be used as adjunctive therapy.

Several medications have been used for acute migraine treatment including analgesics, antiemetics, anxiolytics, nonsteroidal antiinflammatory drugs, ergots, steroids, major tranquilizers, and narcotics. Recently, triptans (selective 5-$HT_{1B/D}$ [serotonin] agonists) have been used with success (sumatriptan, rizatriptan, zolmitriptan, naratriptan), and more recently, new options available are eletriptan, almotriptan, and frovatriptan.

Preventive treatments include a broad range of medications, most notably antidepressants, anticonvulsants, serotonin antagonists, β-blockers, and calcium channel blockers. Botulinum toxin type A therapy is a promising alternative.

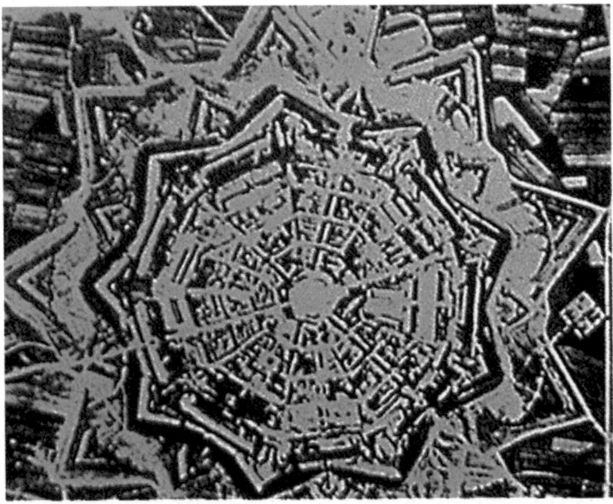

**Figure 5.1** Fortification spectra seen in migraine visual auras have been compared to the aerial view of the fortified, walled city of Palmanova, Italy. Reproduced with permission from Silberstein SD, Lipton RB, Goadsby PJ. *Headache in Clinical Practice*. Oxford: Isis Medical Media, 1998:64

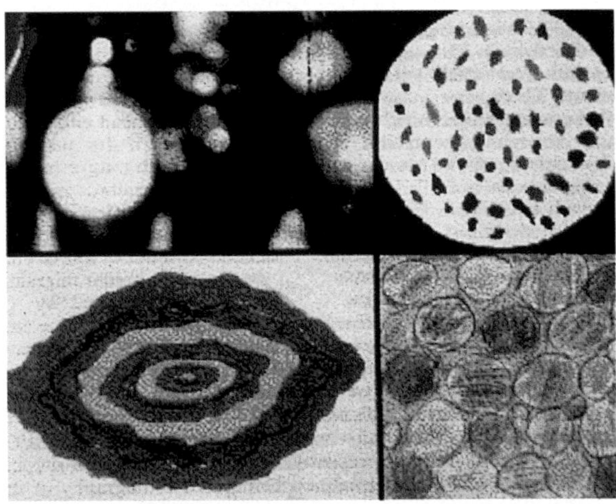

**Figure 5.2** Migraine visual auras are very similar to epileptic visual hallucinations seen here. Reproduced from Panayiotopoulos CP. Elementary visual hallucinations in migraine and epilepsy. *J Neurol Neurosurg Psychiatr* 1994;57: 1371–4, with permission from the BMJ Publishing Group

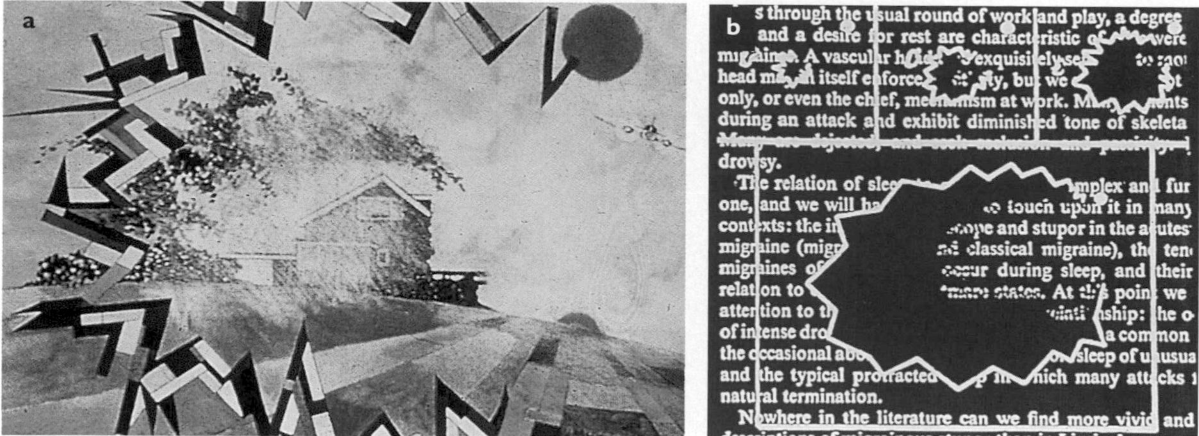

**Figure 5.3** (a) An artist's representation of his visual disturbance during a migraine attack. In this the fortification spectrum is part of a formal design but still maintains a crescentic shape. There is also an associated partial visual loss. (b) An artist's representation similar to one of the images in Sir William Gowers' 1904 paper showing a progressive central scotoma with a jagged edge. The scotoma gradually increases to fill most of the central field. Reproduced with permission from Wilkinson M, Robinson D. Migraine art. *Cephalalgia* 1985;5:151–7

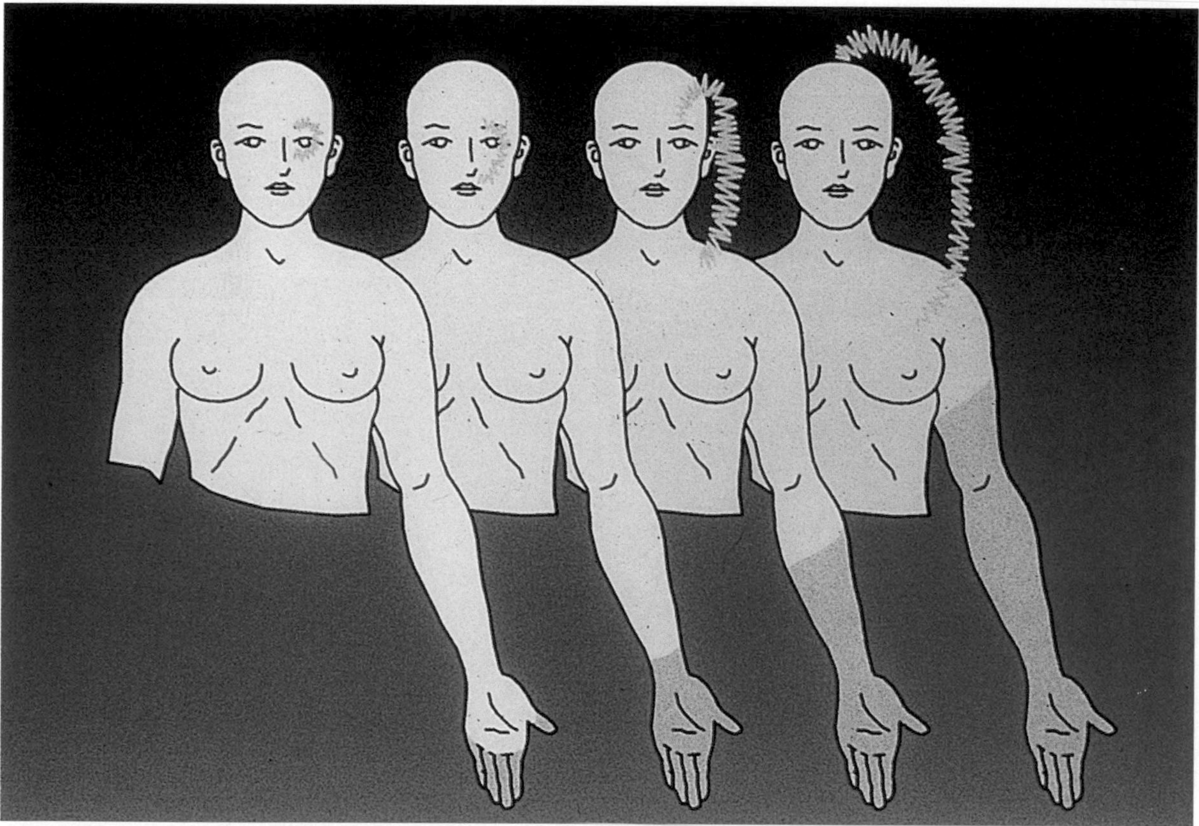

**Figure 5.4** Paresthesias are the second most common migraine aura. Adapted from Spierings ELH. Symptomatology and pathogenesis. In: *Management of Migraine*. Boston, MA: Butterworth-Heinemann, 1996:7–19

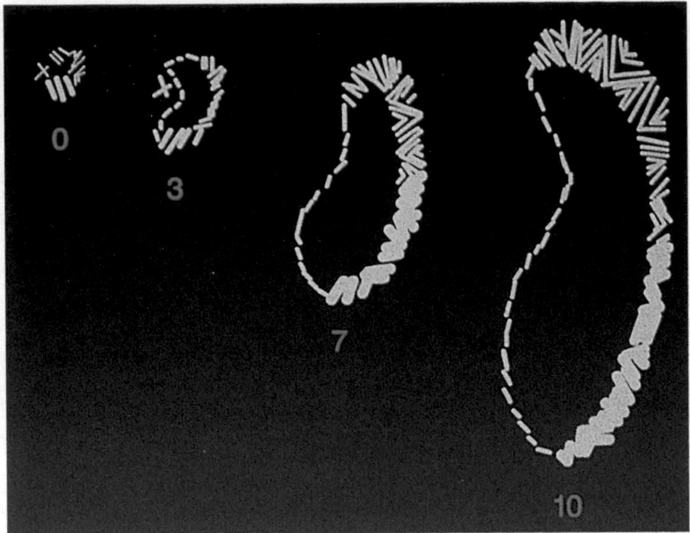


**Figure 5.5** Fortification spectra as depicted by Lashley. An arch of scintillating lights, usually but not always beginning near the point of fixation, may form into a herringbone-like pattern that expands to encompass an increasing portion of the visual hemifield. It migrates across the visual field with a scintillating edge of often zigzag, flashing or occasionally colored phenomena. Reproduced with permission from Lashley K. Patterns of cerebral integration indicated by the scotomas of migraine. *Arch Neurol Psychiatr* 1941;46:331–9

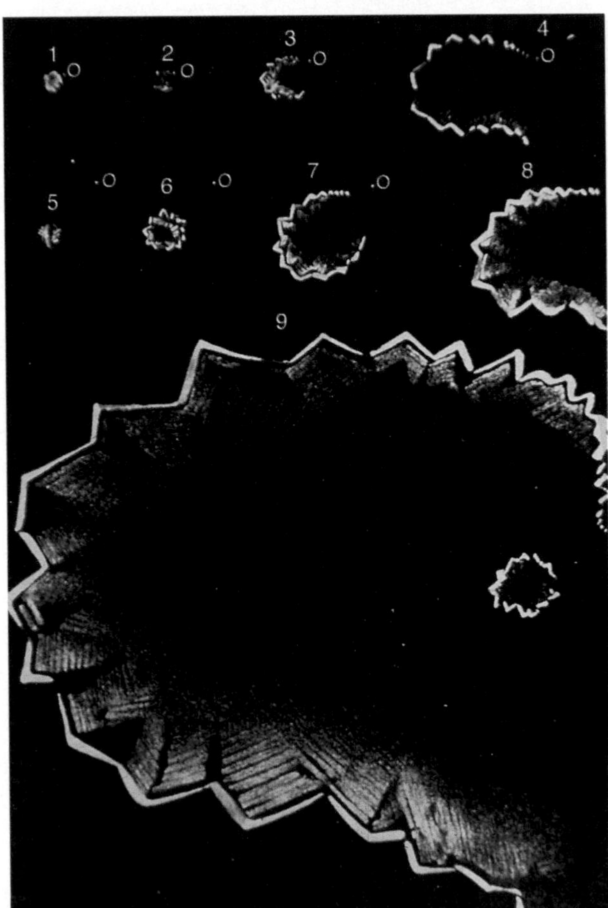


**Figure 5.6** Migraine aura. 1–4, Early stages of sinistral teichopsia beginning close to the sight point, as seen in the dark. The letter O marks the sight point in every figure; 5–8, a similar series of the early stages of sinistral teichopsia beginning a few degrees below and to the left of the sight point; 9, sinistral teichopsia fully developed. Beginning of a secondary attack, which never attains full development, until it arises on the opposite side

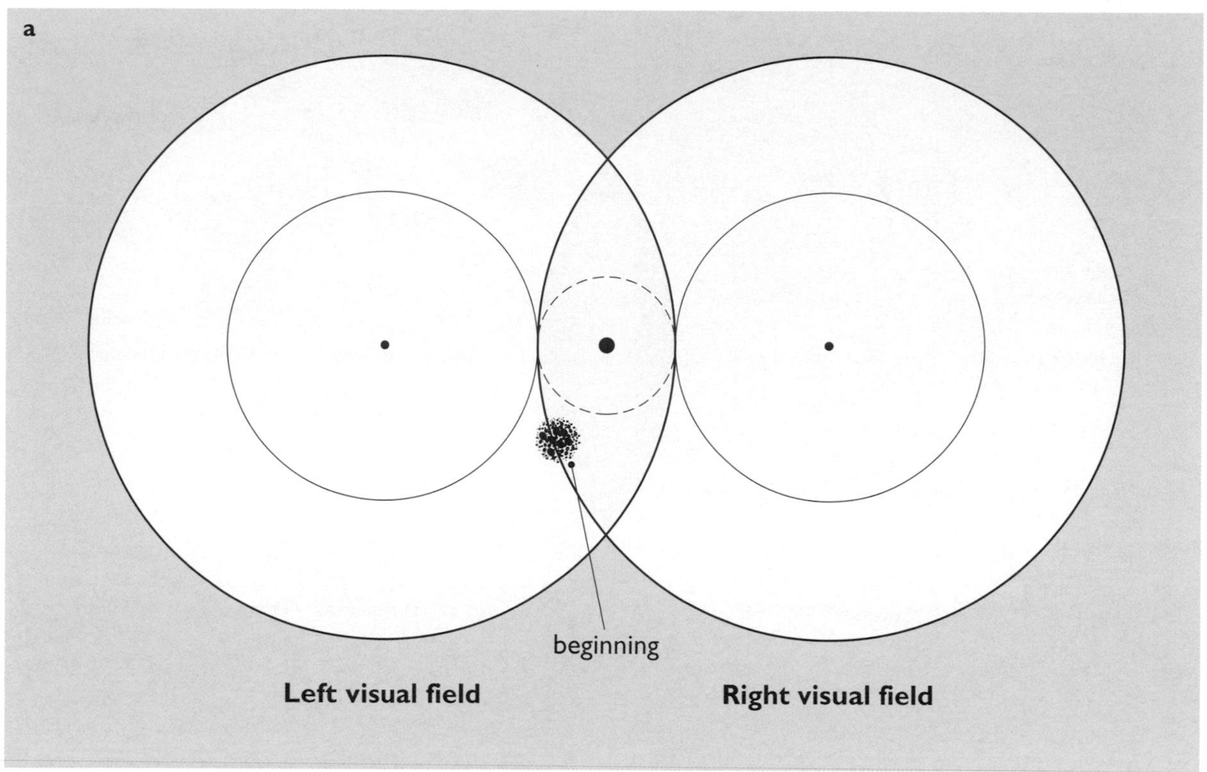


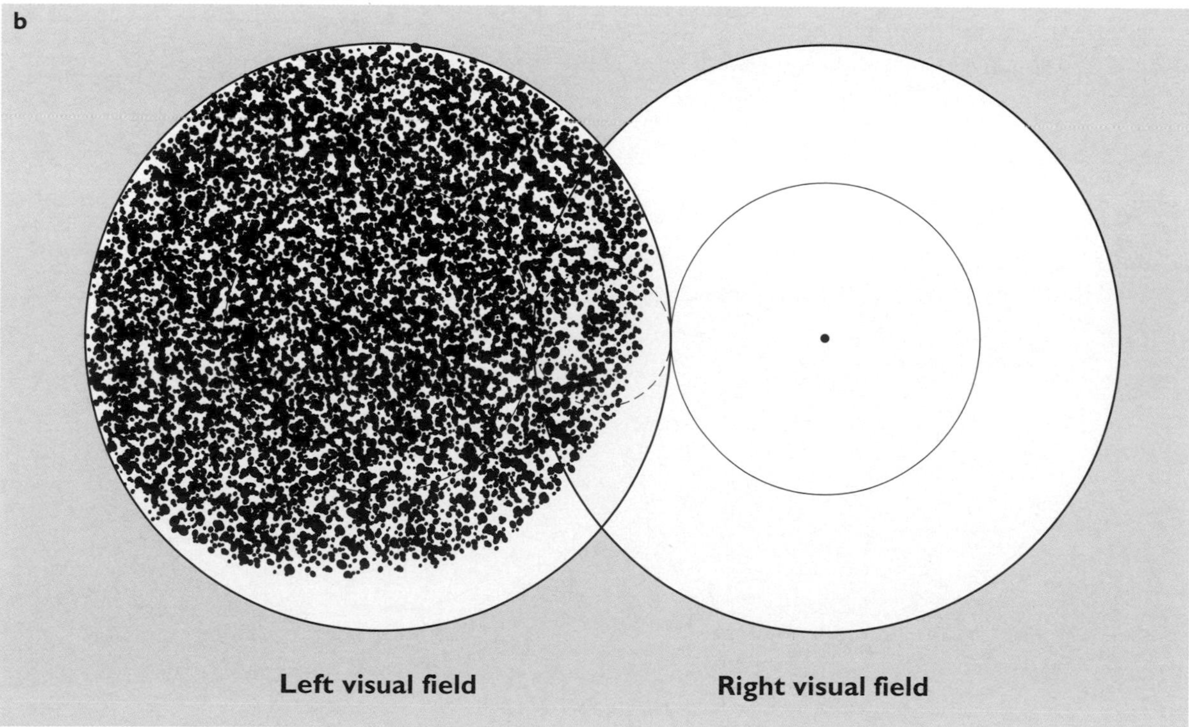


**Figure 5.7** (a) and (b) Adapted from drawings by Professor Leao depicting an expanding hemianopsia as seen by a patient experiencing migraine visual aura, with kind permission of Luiz Paulo de Queiroz

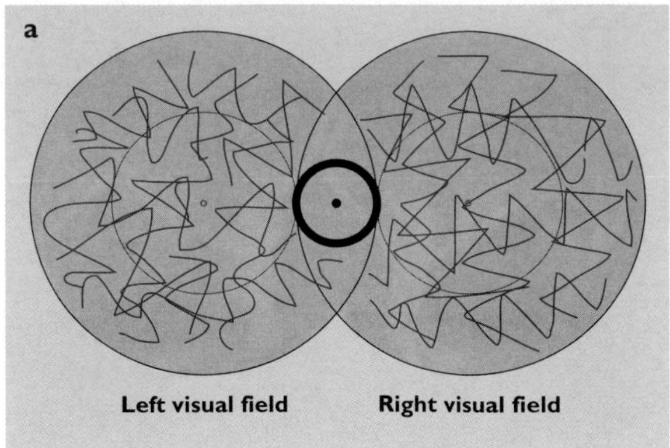


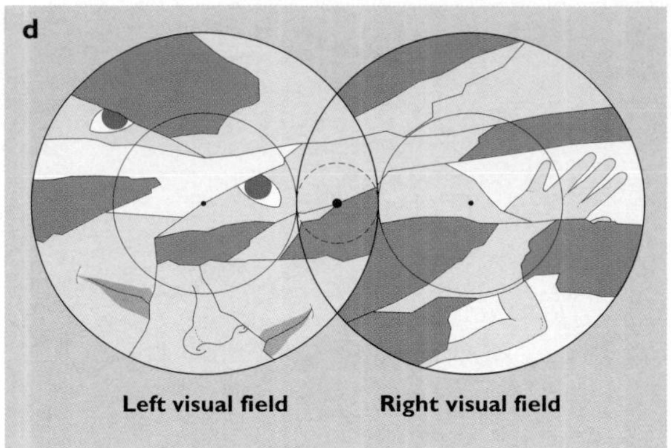


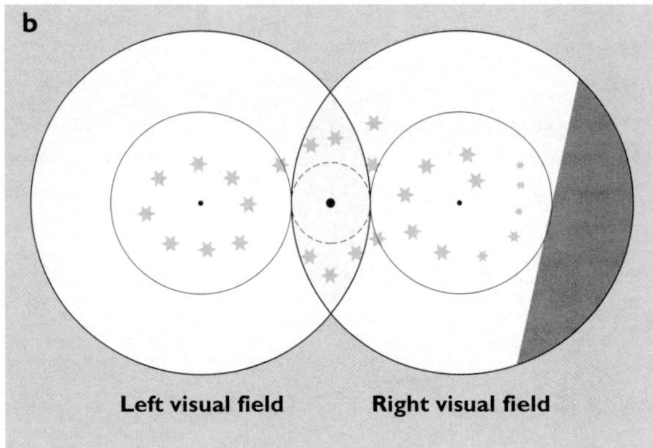


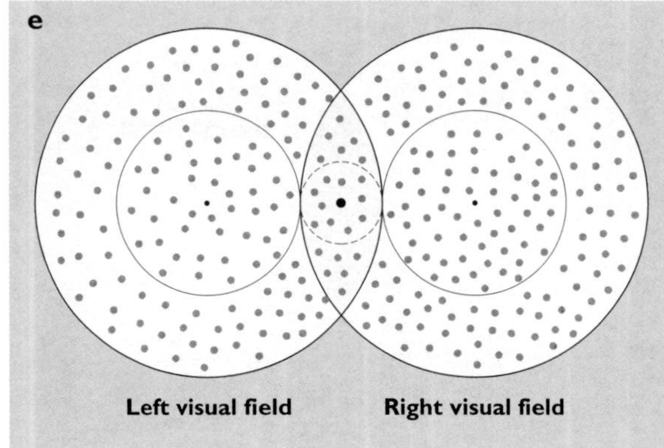


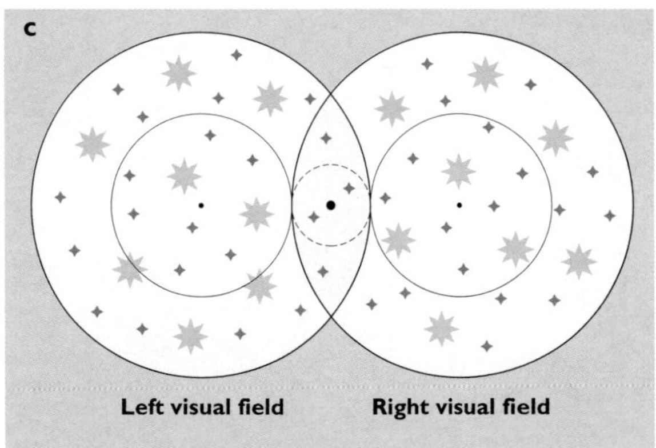


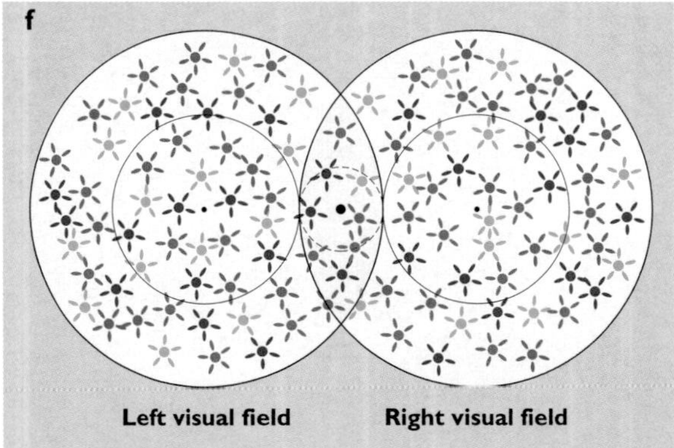


**Figure 5.8** (a) to (f) Adapted from drawings by Professor Leao depicting a variety of visual auras described by patients, with kind permission of Luiz Paulo de Queiroz

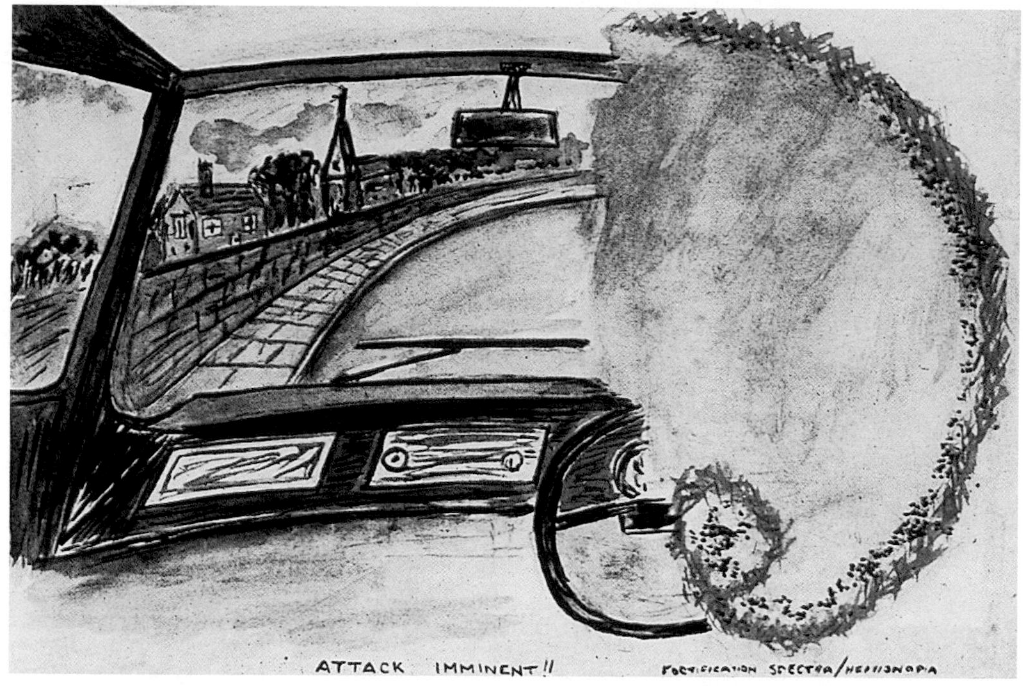


**Figure 5.9** Motorist's right-sided hemianopic loss of vision, the scotomatous area being surrounded by a crescentic area of brighter lights. Reproduced with permission from Wilkinson M, Robinson D. Migraine art. *Cephalalgia* 1985;5:151–7

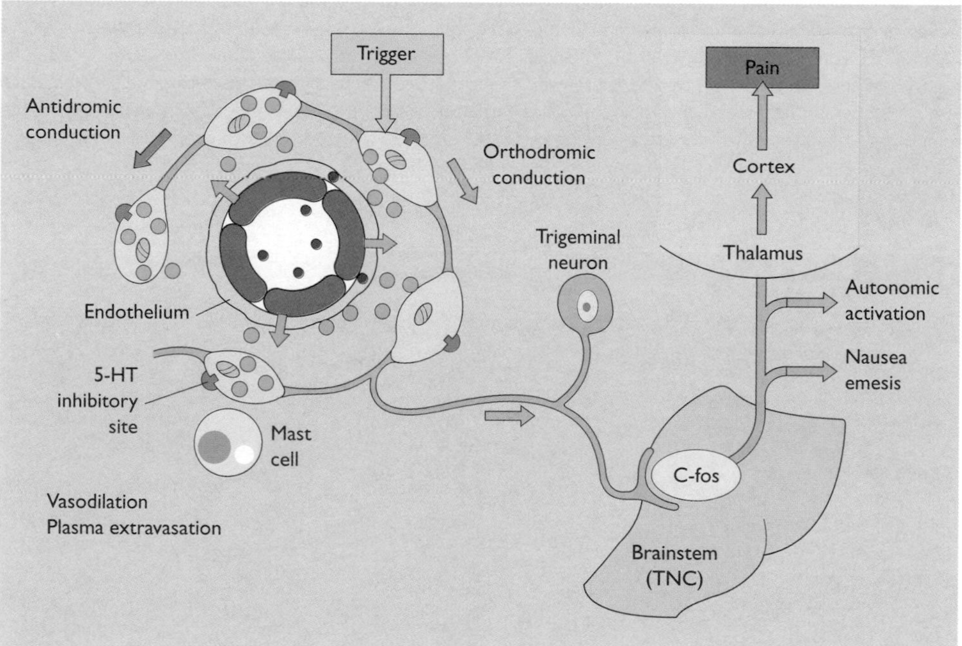


**Figure 5.10** Pathophysiologic mechanism and postulated anti-nociceptive site for sumatriptan and ergot alkaloids in vascular headaches. The triggers for headache activate perivascular trigeminal axons, which release vasoactive neuropeptides to promote neurogenic inflammation (vasodilation, plasma extravasation, mast cell degranulation). Ortho- and antidromic conduction along trigeminovascular fibers spreads the inflammatory response to adjacent tissues and transmits nociceptive information towards the trigeminal nucleus caudalis and higher brain centers for the registration of pain. TNC, trigeminal nucleus caudalis. Adapted from Moskowitz MA. Neurogenic versus vascular mechanisms of sumatriptan and ergot alkaloids in migraine. *Trends Pharmacol Sci* 1992;13:307–11, with permission from Elsevier Science

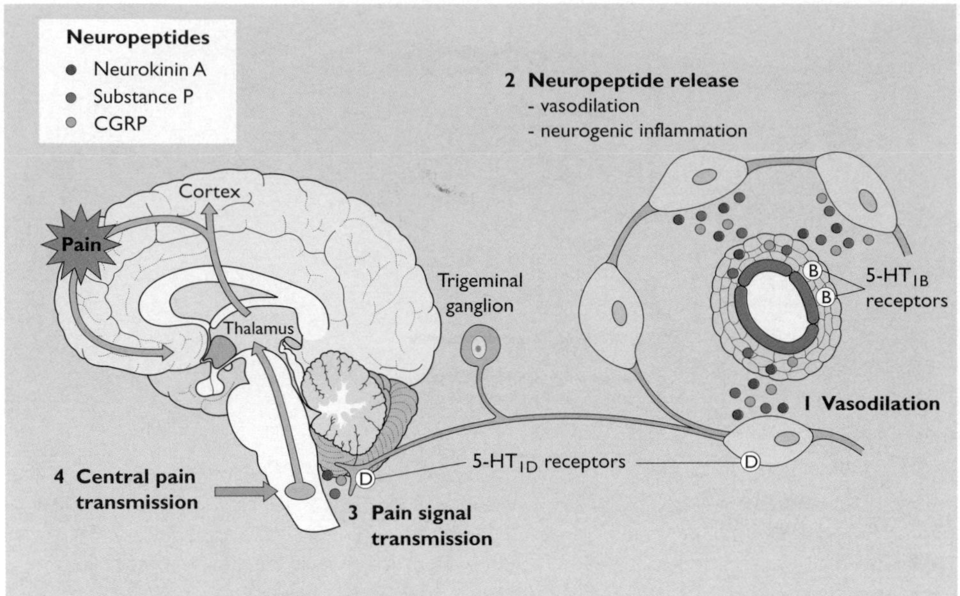


**Figure 5.11** A primary dysfunction of brain stem pain and vascular control centers elicits a cascade of secondary changes in vascular regulation within pain-producing intracranial structures that ultimately manifests in headache pain and associated symptoms. A synthesis of these views and observations forms the neurovascular hypothesis of migraine. It is critical to understand the anatomy of the trigeminal vascular system and the pathophysiologic events that arise during a migraine attack before considering the proposed mechanisms of action of acute therapies. Current theories suggest that there are several key steps in the generation of migraine pain: (**1**) Intracranial meningeal blood vessel dilation which activates perivascular sensory trigeminal nerves. (**2**) Vasoactive neuropeptide release from activated trigeminal sensory nerves. These peptides can worsen and perpetuate any existing vasodilation, setting up a vicious cycle that increases sensory nerve activation and intensifies headache pain. The peptides include substance P (increased vascular permeability), neurokinin A (dilation and permeability changes) and calcitonin gene-related peptide (CGRP; long-lasting vasodilation). (**3**) Pain impulses from activated peripheral sensory nerves are relayed to second-order sensory neurons within the trigeminal nucleus caudalis in the brain stem and upper cervical spinal cord (C1 and C2, trigeminocervical complex). (**4**) Headache pain signals ascend to the thalamus, via the quintothalamic tract which decussates in the brain stem, and on to higher cortical centers where migraine pain is registered and perceived. Adapted with permission from Hargreaves RJ, Shepheard SL. Pathophysiology of migraine – new insights. *Can J Neurol Sci* 1999;26(Suppl 3):S12–19

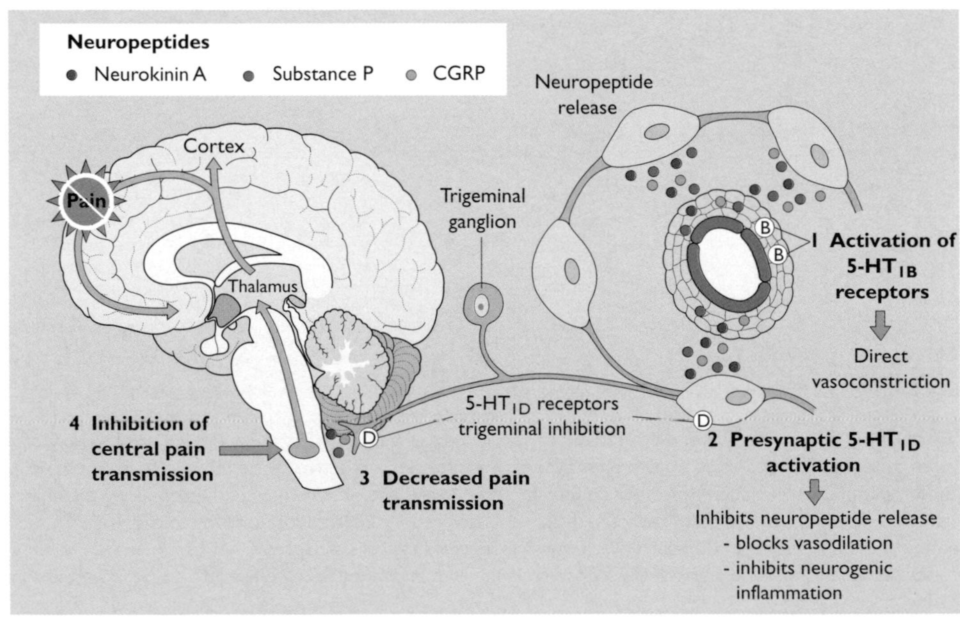

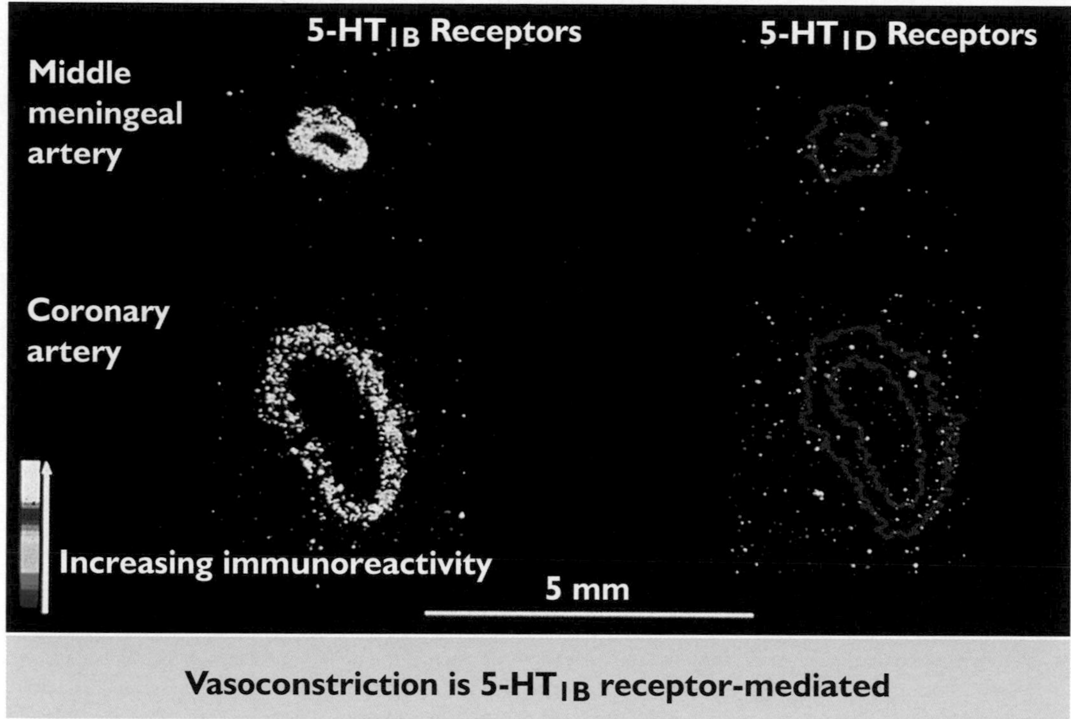


**Figure 5.13** 5-$HT_{1B/1D}$ receptor immunoreactivity in human cranial and coronary arteries. The left column reveals positive immunofluorescence consistent with the presence of 5-$HT_{1B}$ receptors on the blood vessels, while the right column shows negative staining for 5-$HT_{1D}$ receptors. Therefore, it is the agonist effect at 5-$HT_{1B}$ receptors that results in vasoconstriction. Reproduced with permission from Longmore J, Razzaque Z, Shaw D, *et al*. Comparison of the vasoconstrictor effects of rizatriptan and sumatriptan in human isolated cranial arteries: immunohistochemical demonstration of the involvement of 5-$HT_{1B}$ receptors. *Br J Clin Pharmacol* 1998;46:577–82

**Figure 5.12** *(opposite)* Increased knowledge of 5-HT receptor distribution within the trigeminovascular system has led to the introduction of highly effective serotonergic anti-migraine drug therapies. Detailed molecular biology mapping of mRNA (RT-PCR and *in situ* hybridization) and immunohistochemical studies of recepter proteins have revealed populations of vasoconstrictor 5-$HT_{1B}$ receptors on the smooth muscle of human meningeal blood vessels. Thus, agonists of 5-$HT_{1B}$ receptors, which cause vasoconstriction, are ideally placed to reverse the dilation of meningeal vessels that is thought to occur during a migraine attack (see **1**). 5-$HT_{1B}$ receptors have also been found on human coronary arteries making it important to establish the relative contribution of this subtype to the contractile response in coronary arteries compared with the target meningeal blood vessels. While 5-$HT_{1F}$ mRNA has also been demonstrated in human blood vessels, there appears to be no expression of functional receptors since 5-$HT_{1F}$ agonists appear devoid of vasoconstrictor effects. Immunohistochemical mapping studies on the localization of 5-$HT_{1D}$ and 5-$HT_{1F}$ receptor proteins in human trigeminal nerves have shown that 5-$HT_{1D}$ and 5-$HT_{1F}$ receptors are present on trigeminal nerves projecting peripherally to the dural vasculature and centrally to the brain stem trigeminal nuclei. Activation of such prejunctional receptors on nerve terminals can modulate neurotransmitter release. In this context, agonists of 5-$HT_{1D}$ and 5-$HT_{1F}$ receptors are ideally placed, peripherally (see **2**) to inhibit activated trigeminal nerves and promote normalization of blood vessel caliber (by preventing the release of vasoactive neuropeptides) and centrally (see **3**) to intercept pain signal transmission from the meningeal blood vessels to second-order sensory neurons in the trigeminal nucleus caudalis of the brain stem (see **4**). Adapted with permission from Hargreaves RJ, Shepheard SL. Pathophysiology of migraine – new insights. *Can J Neurol Sci* 1999;26(Suppl 3):S12–19

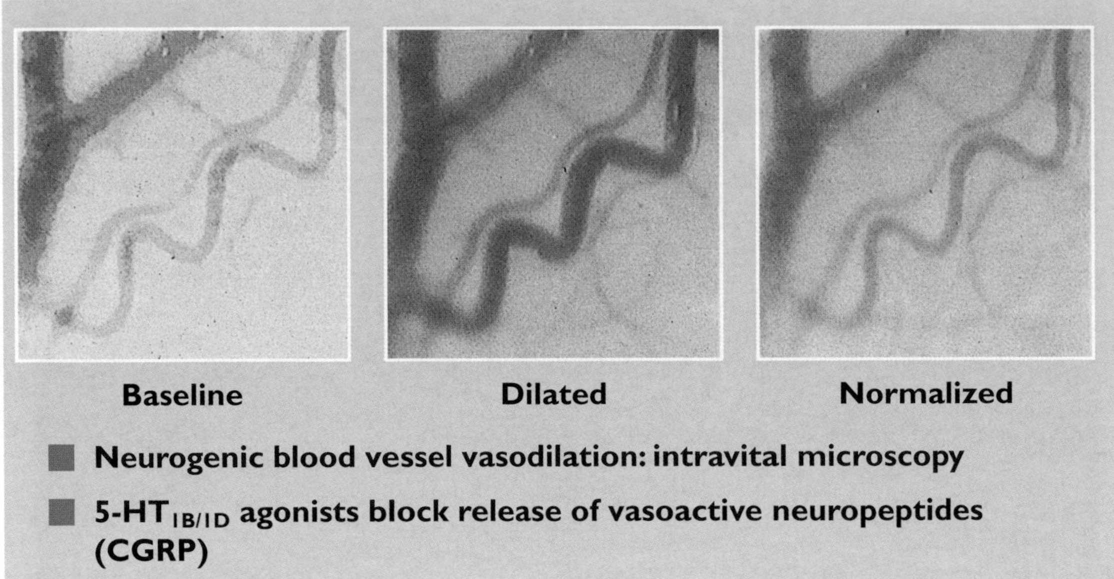


**Figure 5.14** Results from a preclinical intravital microscope dural plasma protein extravasation (DPPE) assay that was used to investigate the anti-migraine action of rizatriptan. These videoframes show a branch of the middle meningeal artery embedded within the dura mater (running bottom left to top right of each section). The sequence shows the artery at baseline (left panel), in a dilated state after electrically evoked vasoactive neuropeptide release from the perivascular nerves (middle panel) and when normalized by drug treatment.

These intravital studies showed that rizatriptan blocks the electrically evoked release of peptides including CGRP from perivascular sensory nerves in the meninges but does not inhibit vessel dilation to CGRP when it is given intravenously. This suggests that rizatriptan is not a CGRP receptor antagonist but instead inhibits the release of CGRP from trigeminal sensory nerves. This blockade of neuropeptide release is thought to occur through stimulation of prejunctional 5-$HT_{1D}$ receptors. Since all of the 5-$HT_{1B/1D}$ agonists are capable of blocking the release of vasoactive neuropeptides, it suggests that one mechanism of action of these drugs is blockade of neurogenic inflammation. Reproduced with permission from Shepheard SL, Williamson DJ, Hargreaves RJ. Intravital microscope studies of dural blood vessels in rats. In: *Migraine and Headache Pathophysiology*, 1st edn. London: Martin Dunitz, 1999:103–17

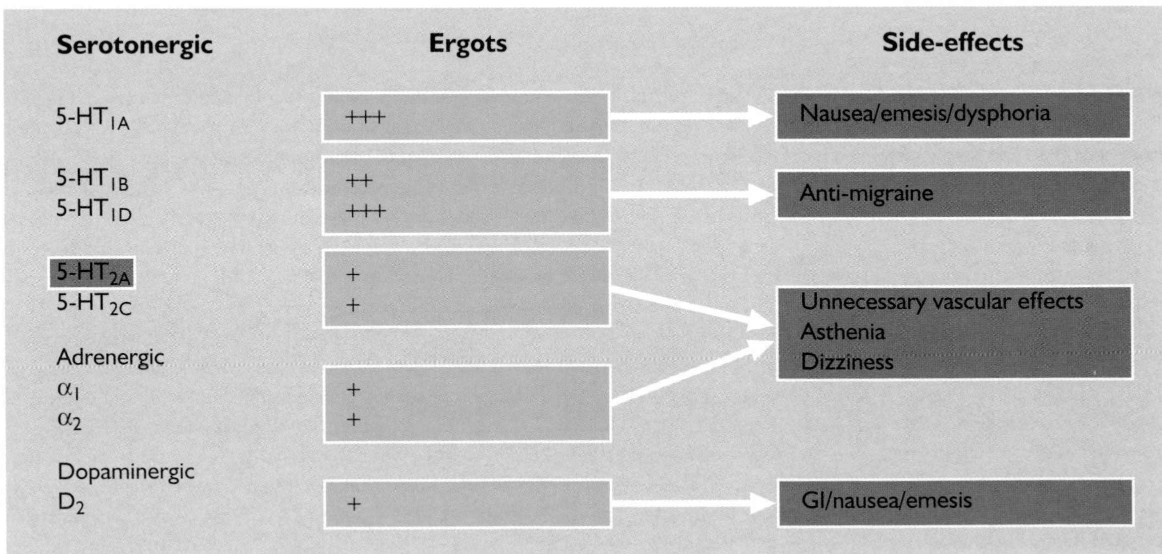

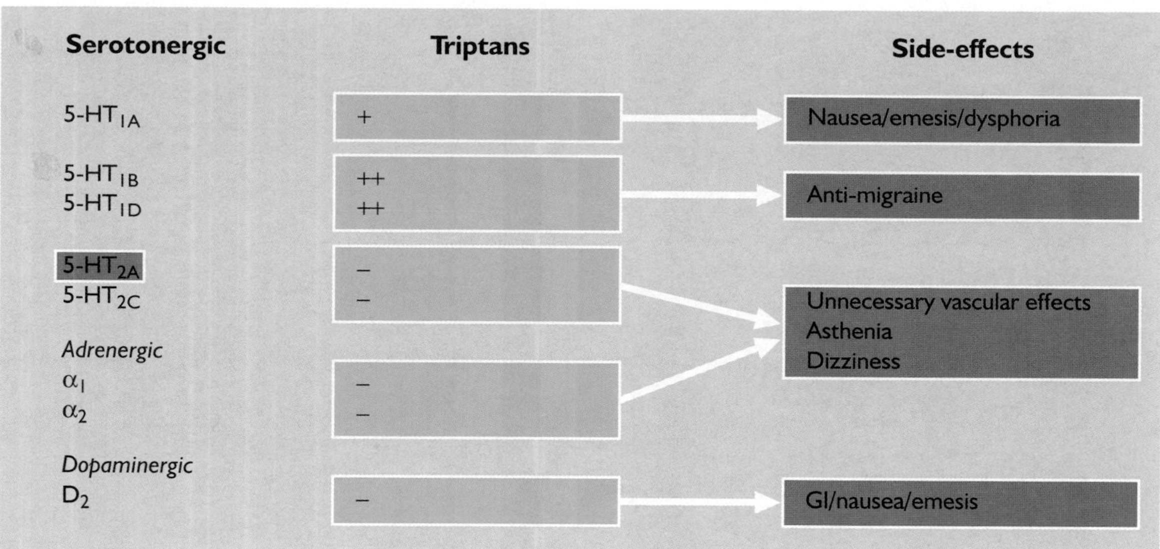


**Figure 5.16** The triptans selectively target and activate $5\text{-HT}_{1B}$ and $5\text{-HT}_{1D}$ receptors. Like the ergots, they have potent activity at the 'anti-migraine' $5\text{-HT}_{1B/1D}$ receptors but have much weaker action at $5\text{-HT}_{1A}$ receptors. The triptans lack binding activity on the monoamine receptors of the ergots. Adapted from Goadsby PJ. Serotonin $5\text{-HT}_{1B/1D}$ receptor antagonists in migraine. *CNS Drugs* 1998;10:271–86

**Figure 5.15** *(opposite)* The ergots were the first 5-HT agonists used for the treatment of migraine. They are not particularly useful when given orally due to their unpredictable absorption and their low bioavailability. This is improved, however, by intranasal or rectal administration. The peripheral vascular effects of the ergots were already known during the Middle Ages, when they caused the disorder known as 'Saint Anthony's fire' due to the ingestion of bread infected by *Claviceps purpurea*, the ergot-producing fungus (see Chapter 1). This caused such a profound vasoconstriction of the extremities that patients felt as if their extremities were burning with the latter eventually turning black. The victims looked as if they had been charred by fire and the epidemic got its name from this fact. Nausea and dizziness, the common side-effects of ergots, may be explained by the actions of these compounds on multiple monoamine receptors.

Ergots are potent agonists at the $5\text{-HT}_{1B/1D}$ receptors and this explains their anti-migraine effect. They also act on $5\text{-HT}_{1A}$ receptors, an activation that is probably responsible for the production of nausea and dysphoria. The constriction of the peripheral vasculature is probably through activation of α-adrenoreceptors and $5\text{-HT}_{2A}$ receptors. Agonist activity at dopamine $D_2$ receptors produces gastrointestinal disturbances, nausea and emesis. Thus, based on their pharmacologic activity at monoamine receptors, it is possible to conclude that although ergots are good anti-migraine agents, they also have many other unwanted effects. Adapted from Goadsby PJ. Serotonin $5\text{-HT}_{1B/1D}$ receptor antagonists in migraine. *CNS Drugs* 1998;10:271–86

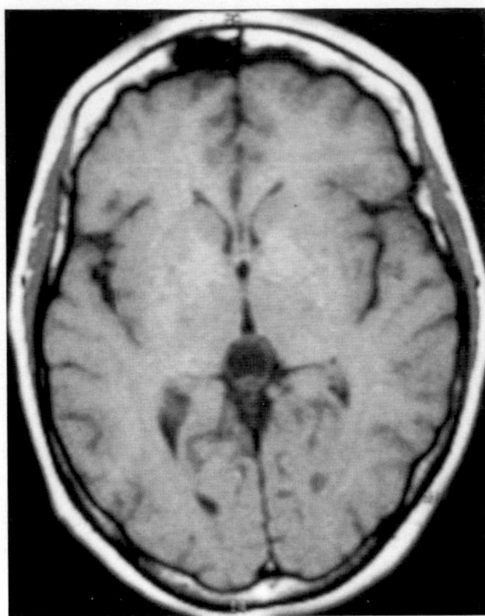

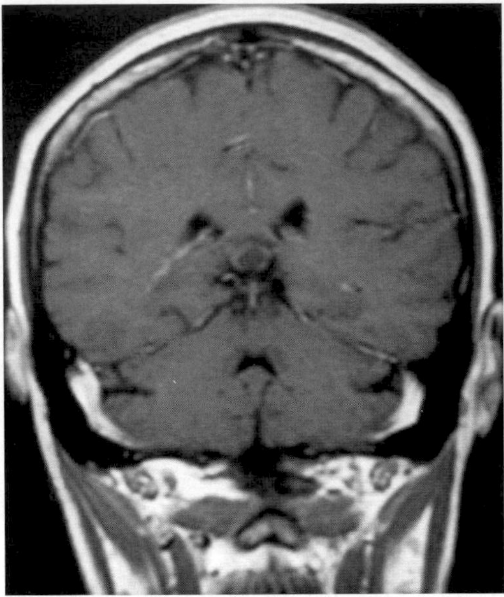

**Figure 5.17** This is a 37-year-old right-handed women with a history of 11 years of headaches, transformed to daily frequency in the past 2 years. The patient was diagnosed with chronic migraine. Her neurological examination disclosed abnormalities. Brain MRI (axial and coronal T1 weighted) showed a pineal cyst; in the follow-up, cyst size did not change

# 6

# Trigeminal-autonomic cephalgias

Todd D Rozen

## INTRODUCTION

This chapter will discuss the distinct headache disorders known as the trigeminal-autonomic cephalgias (TACs). This group of primary headaches is characterized by short-duration unilateral head pains and associated ipsilateral autonomic symptoms. Recognized TACs include cluster headache, chronic paroxysmal hemicrania (CPH), episodic paroxysmal hemicrania (EPH) and the syndrome of short-lasting unilateral neuralgiform headache with conjunctival injection and tearing (SUNCT) (Table 6.1). Cluster headache is a fairly common condition, while CPH and SUNCT may never be seen by physicians in their entire practice lifetime. What sets these headaches apart from the other primary headache disorders, such as migraine and tension-type headache, is the extreme intensity of the headache and the unique associated symptoms representing both parasympathetic nervous system activation (eye lacrimation, conjunctival injection, nasal congestion or rhinorrhea) and sympathetic nervous system dysfunction (miosis, ptosis, partial Horner's syndrome). What distinguishes each of the TACs from each other is the duration of the headache attacks. SUNCT has the shortest duration, with attacks lasting 5–240 s (Figure 6.1). CPH attacks last 2–30 min (Figure 6.2) and cluster headaches attacks last 15–180 min (Figure 6.3). What ties the syndromes together is a linkage between headache and autonomic symptoms. This clinical phenotype can be explained by an underlying trigeminal-autonomic reflex pathway which consists

**Table 6.1** The differential diagnosis for cluster headache involves the other known trigeminal-autonomic cephalgias: SUNCT, CPH, EPH, idiopathic stabbing headache and trigeminal neuralgia. Based on individual attack duration, attack frequency and associated symptoms, a correct diagnosis of cluster can be made. In the United States it takes an average of six years before a cluster patient is correctly diagnosed. It should not be difficult to make a diagnosis of cluster if a good headache history is taken. PPT, precipitant. Reproduced with permission from reference 1

| *Feature* | *Cluster* | *CPH* | *EPH* | *SUNCT* | *Stabbing headache* | *Trigeminal neuralgia* |
|---|---|---|---|---|---|---|
| Gender (M:F) | 4:1 | 1:3 | 1:1 | 2.3:1 | F > M | F > M |
| Attack duration | 15–180 min | 2–30 min | 1–30 min | 5–240 s | < 1 s | < 1 s |
| Attack frequency | 1–8/day | 1–40/day | 3–30/day | 1/day–30/h | Few–many | Few–many |
| Autonomic features | + | + | + | + | – | – |
| Alcohol PPT | + | + | + | + | – | – |
| Indomethacin effect | +/– | + | + | – | + | – |

of a brainstem connection between the trigeminal nerve and the facial nerve and the facial nerve (the site of the cranial parasympathetic outflow system). It is very important to the clinician to recognize the TACs as distinct headache disorders outside of migraine and tension-type headache, because treatment strategies are different for each headache. For example, CPH is an indomethacin-responsive headache syndrome, while cluster headache and SUNCT do not respond to this non-steroidal antiinflammatory agent. In the following paragraphs short descriptions of the distinct TACs will be given. Also, a pictorial presentation of the TACs will be made including images on epidemiology, pathogenesis, clinical characteristics and treatment strategies (Figures 6.1–6.35).

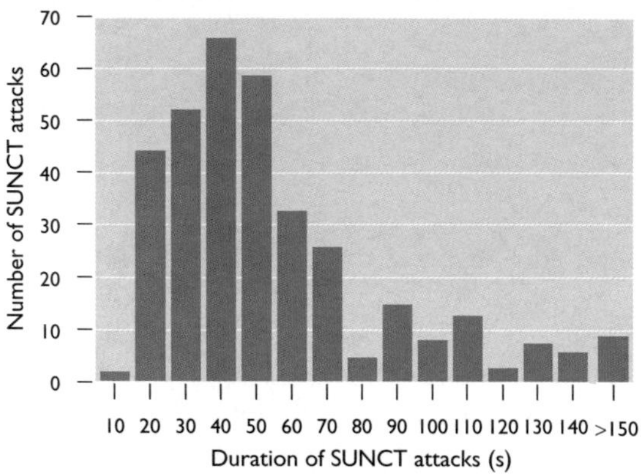


**Figure 6.1** SUNCT is marked by very short-lasting attacks (5 to 240 s) of headache and associated autonomic symptoms. Adapted with permission from Pareja JA, Shen JM, Kruszewski P, *et al.* SUNCT syndrome: duration, frequency, and temporal distribution of attacks. *Headache* 1996;36:161–5

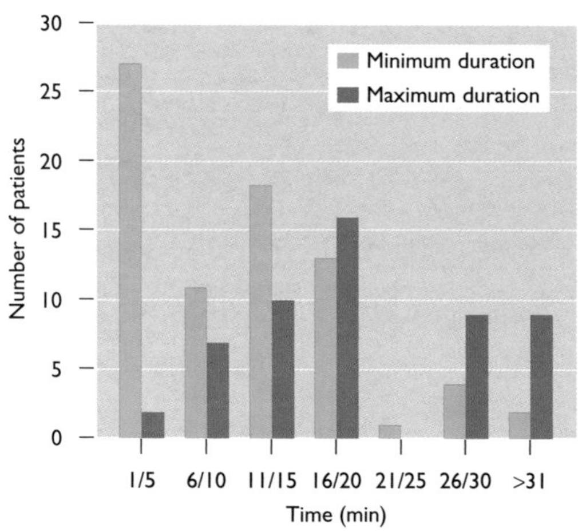


**Figure 6.2** Duration of individual attacks of chronic paroxysmal hemicrania (CPH) in minutes. Most attacks will be 15 to 20 min in duration. Adapted with permission from Antonaci F, Sjaastad O. Chronic paroxysmal hemicrania (CPH): a review of the clinical manifestations. *Headache* 1989;29: 648–56

## CLUSTER HEADACHES

There is no more severe pain than that sustained by a cluster headache sufferer. Cluster headache is known as the 'suicide headache' (for other names of this condition, see Table 6.2), and if not for the rather short duration of attacks most cluster sufferers would

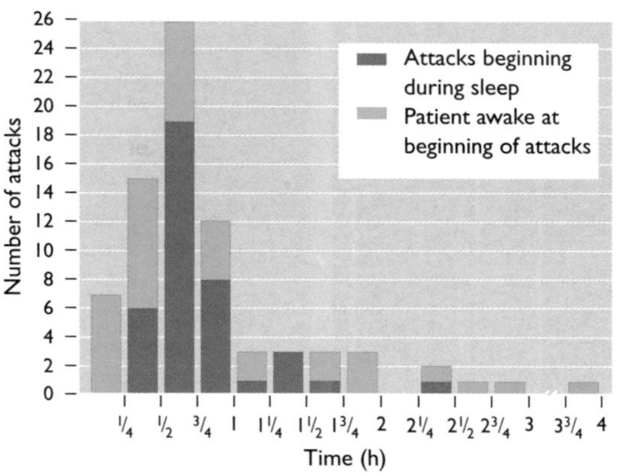


**Figure 6.3** Duration of cluster attacks. Typical attack duration is 1 h or less. Adapted with permission from Russell D. Cluster headache: Severity and temporal profiles of attacks and patient activity prior to and during attacks. *Cephalalgia* 1981;1:209–16

**Table 6.2** Cluster headache has been recognized in the literature by many names, some of which are still used today

| |
|---|
| Hemicrania angioparalytica (Eulenberg, 1878) |
| Sluder's sphenopalatine neuralgia (Sluder, 1908) |
| Ciliary neuralgia, migrainous neuralgia (Harris, 1926) |
| Autonomic faciocephalalgia (Brickner and Riley, 1935) |
| Erythromelalgia of the head, histaminic cephalalgia (Horton, 1939, 1941; Figure 6.11) |

choose death rather than continue suffering. Cluster headache is a primary headache syndrome (Figure 6.4). It is very stereotyped in its presentation and fairly easy to diagnose with an in-depth headache history. Fortunately cluster headaches are easy to treat in most individuals if the correct medications are used and the correct dosages given. Our understanding of the pathogenesis of cluster headaches is increasing, and this should lead to better and more specific cluster therapies. Recently Klapper *et al.*[2] determined that the average time it takes for a cluster sufferer to be diagnosed correctly by the medical profession is 6.6 years. This statistic is unacceptable based on the pain and suffering cluster patients must endure when they are not treated correctly or not treated at all. In many instances cluster headache is misdiagnosed as migraine or sinus headache, so an inappropriate therapy regime is prescribed. In 2004, the International Headache Society (IHS) revised the diagnostic criteria for cluster headache[3] (Table 6.3). Patients with cluster headache should experience at least five attacks of severe, unilateral, orbital, supraorbital and/or temporal pain that lasts from 15 to 180 min untreated. The headache needs to be associated with at least one of the following signs or symptoms: lacrimation, conjunctival injection, rhinorrhea, nasal congestion, forehead and facial sweating, miosis, ptosis or eyelid edema (Table 6.4). Cluster headaches are typically side-fixed and will remain on the same side of the head for a patient's entire lifetime. Only 15% of patients will have a shift of sides between

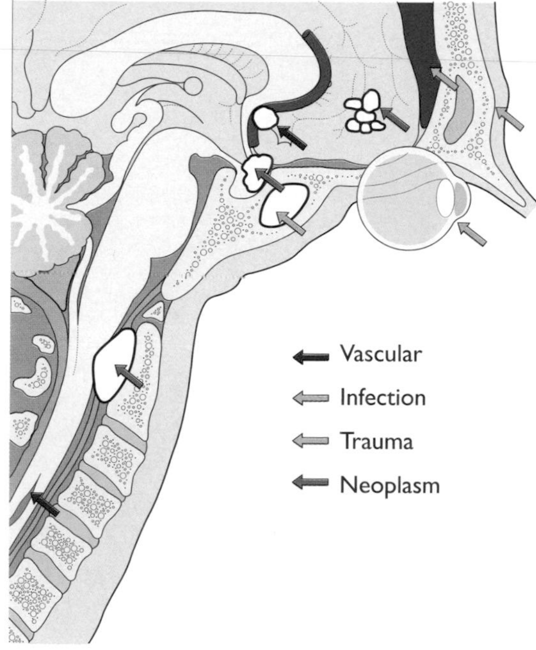


**Figure 6.4** Cluster headache is considered a primary headache disorder, so there are no underlying secondary causes. In rare instances cluster headache has been linked to various secondary causes including: aneurysms, head trauma, orbital enucleation, sphenoid sinusitis, parasellar tumors, cervical cord mengiomas or infarction, subdural hematomas and arteriovenous malformations. Adapted from the Neurology Ambassador Program with permission from the American Headache Society

**Table 6.3** International Headache Society's classification of cluster headache. Adapted with permission from reference 3

| Diagnostic criteria: |
|---|
| A. At least five attacks fulfilling criteria B–D |
| B. Severe or very severe unilateral orbital, supraorbital and/or temporal pain lasting 15–180 min if untreated |
| C. Headache is accompanied by at least one of the following:<br>1. ipsilateral conjunctival injection and/or lacrimation<br>2. ipsilateral nasal congestion and/or rhinorrhea<br>3. ipsilateral eyelid edema<br>4. ipsilateral forehead and facial sweating<br>5. ipsilateral miosis and/or ptosis<br>6. a sense of restlessness or agitation |
| D. Attacks have a frequency from one every other day to 8 per day |
| E. Not attributed to another disorder |

**Table 6.4** Distribution of associated symptoms with cluster headaches. Lacrimation is the most common symptom. Cluster patients do get 'migrainous associated symptoms'. If a cluster patient has typical cluster symptoms but also has nausea and vomiting, the diagnosis is still cluster and not migraine

| *Autonomic symptoms* |
|---|
| Lacrimation (73%) |
| Conjunctival injection (60%) |
| Nasal congestion (42%) |
| Rhinorrhea (22%) |
| Partial Horner's syndrome (16–84%) |
| *General symptoms* |
| Nausea (10–54%; 29%) |
| Vomiting (1–15%; 9%) |
| Photophobia (5–72%) |
| Phonophobia (12–39%) |

cluster periods. The pain of cluster headaches is described as sharp or boring and usually localizes behind the eye. During a cluster attack, patients cannot and do not want to remain still. They typically pace the floor or even bang their heads against the wall to try and alleviate their pain. Cluster headaches are short in duration compared to some of the other primary headaches, usually with an average duration of 45 min to 1 h (Figure 6.3). Cluster patients will frequently have between one and three attacks per day. The headaches have a predilection for the first REM sleep phase, so the cluster patient will awaken with a severe headache 60–90 min after falling asleep (Figure 6.5). Cluster headaches can be of an episodic (greater than one month of headache-free days per year) or chronic (occuring for more than one year without remission or with remissions lasting less than one month) subtype. Between 80–90% of cluster patients have the episodic variety (Figure 6.6). Cluster periods, or the time when patients are experiencing daily cluster attacks, usually last between 2 and 12 weeks and patients can have 1–2 cluster periods per year (Figure 6.7). It is not uncommon for a patient to experience a cluster period at the same time each year. This circadian periodicity suggests a hypothalamic generator for cluster headaches (Figures 6.8–6.9). In regard to age of onset, cluster headaches are a disorder of young

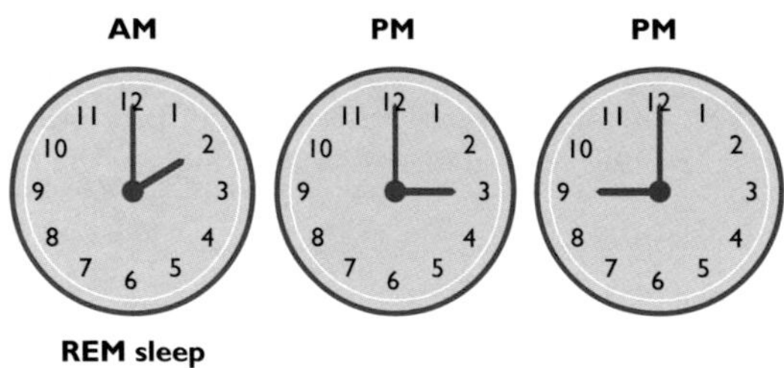


**Figure 6.5** Cluster headache has a distinct circadian periodicity to its attacks. Cluster patients will get attacks at the same time each day and cluster periods at the same time each year. This suggests that the hypothalamus (suprachiasmatic nucleus) or circadian clock is playing a role in cluster genesis. A hallmark of cluster is for the patient to awaken with a cluster headache 1.5 to 2 h after falling asleep (first REM period of the night); typically these night-time attacks are the most painful. Adapted from the Neurology Ambassador Program with permission from the American Headache Society

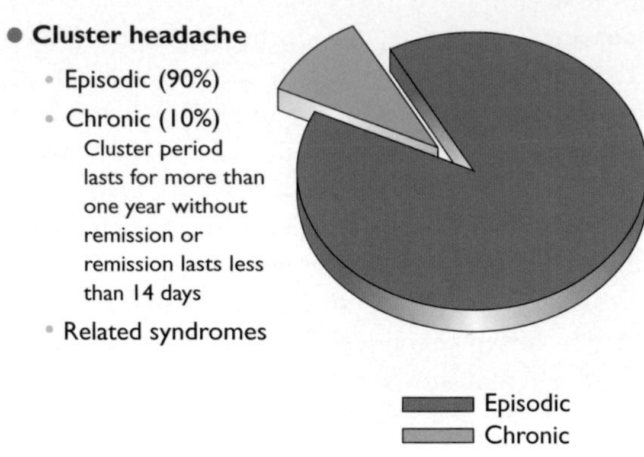


**Figure 6.6** Most cluster patients have the episodic subtype so they will have periods of remission sometimes for years at a time. Adapted from the Neurology Ambassador Program with permission from the American Headache Society

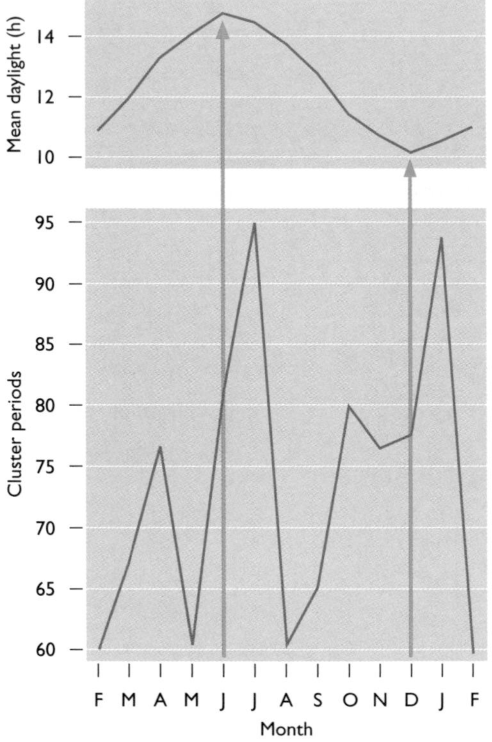


**Figure 6.7** Cluster periods plotted against month of the year and mean monthly daylight duration. Cluster periods appear to occur during the longest and shortest days of the years. Adapted with permission from Kudrow L. The cyclic relationship of natural illumination to cluster period frequency. *Cephalalgia* 1987;7(Suppl 6):76–8

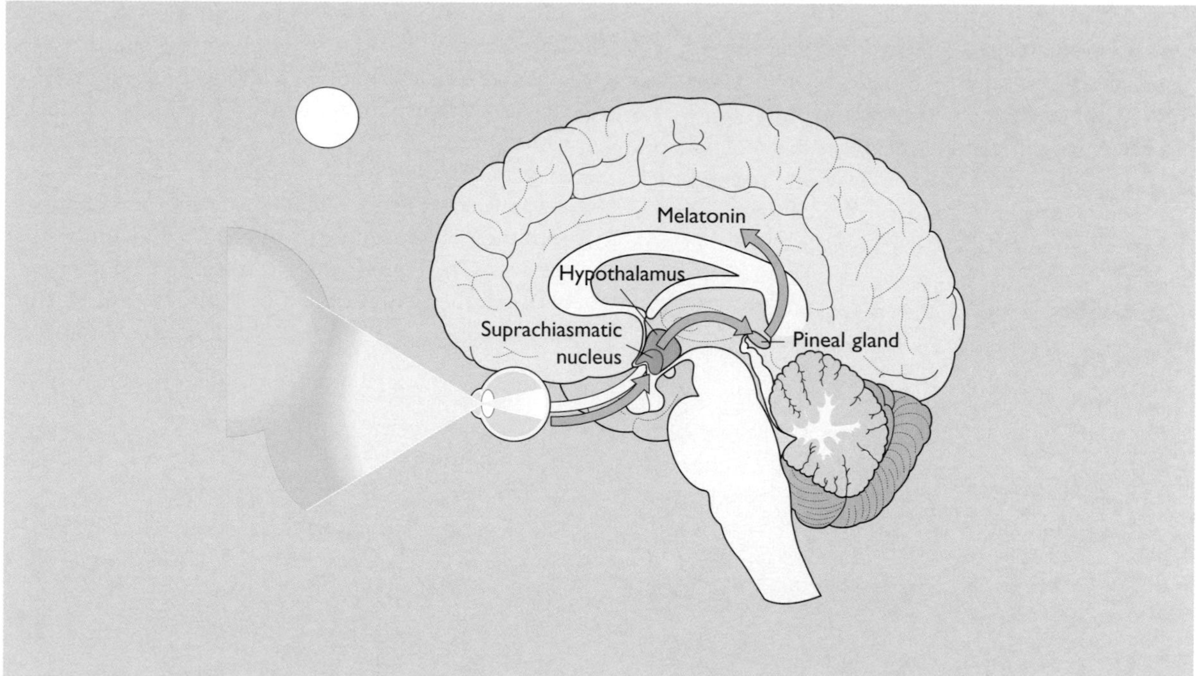


**Figure 6.8** The hypothalamus or circadian clock must be involved in cluster genesis. Cluster headaches have a circannual and circadian rhythmicity, a seasonal predilection for cluster periods and there is altered secretion of hypothalamic hormones in cluster patients (testosterone, melatonin). Adapted from the Neurology Ambassador Program with permission from the American Headache Society

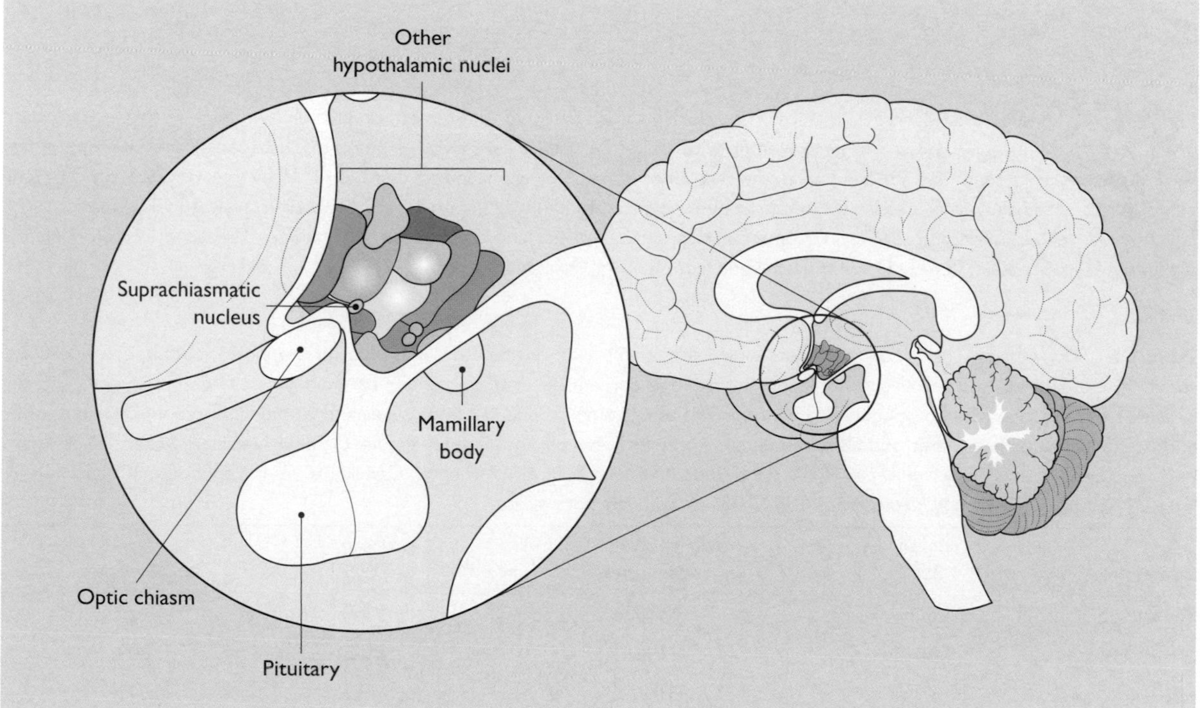


**Figure 6.9** The suprachiasmatic nucleus is the human circadian clock

people but the headaches do not start as young as they do in migraine. Typically cluster headaches will begin in the twenties or thirties, although they can start in the teens or even younger. Men appear to have one age peak of cluster onset in their twenties (Figure 6.10a), while women have one peak in their late teens and twenties and a second in their fifties or sixties (Figure 6.10b). In most instances cluster headaches should be easy to distinguish from migraine based upon the duration of individual attacks (cluster headaches last 15 min to 3 h versus migraines which last > 4 h) and the number of attacks experienced per day (cluster: one or more; migraine: none or one). In addition, only about 3% of cluster patients can remain still during a headache, while almost all migraineurs want to lie down with a migraine. It used to be thought that cluster patients did not experience 'migrainous symptoms' (nausea, vomiting, photophobia, phonophobia) and that these were good distinguishing characteristics between the two disorders, but this may not be true. Photophobia and phonophobia occur almost as

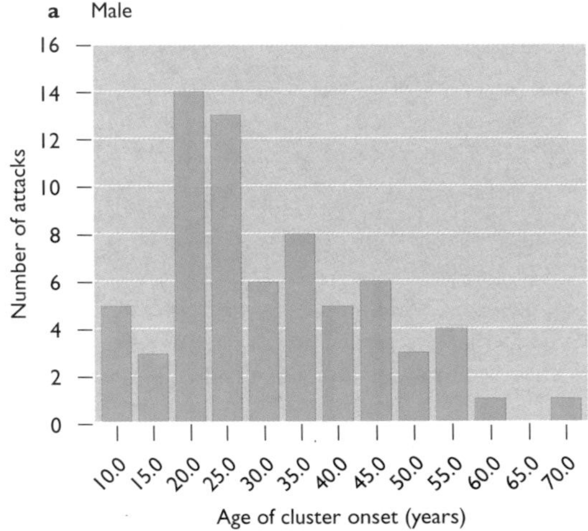


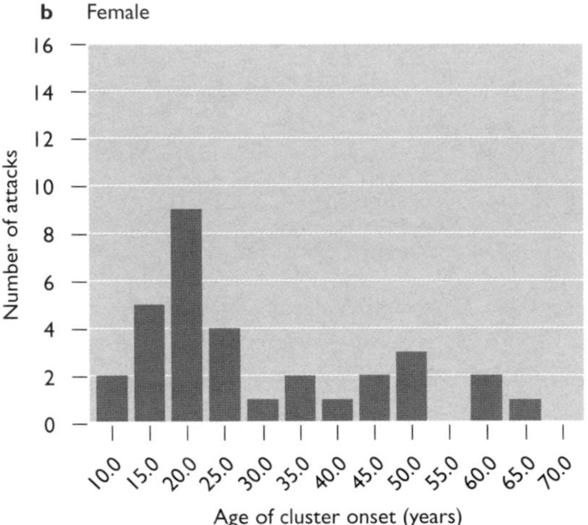


**Figure 6.10** Age of cluster onset. (a) Most men develop their first ever cluster attack in their twenties or thirties (standard deviation = 13.47, mean = 31.3, *n* = 69); (b) women with cluster headaches have two age peaks of cluster onset (unlike men), one in their late teens or twenties and a second when they are 50 or 60 years of age (standard deviation = 15.89, mean = 29.4, *n* = 32). Late age of onset of female cluster headaches needs to be recognized by the treating physician. Adapted from Rozen TD, Niknam RM, Shechter AL, *et al.* Cluster headache in women: clinical characteristics and comparison with cluster headache in men. *J Neurol Neurosurg Psychiatr* 2001;70:613–17, with permission from the BMJ Publishing Group

**Table 6.5** Comparison chart looking at percentage of patients with migrainous symptoms (photophobia, phonophobia, nausea, vomiting) from three cluster investigations and the average percentage of these symptoms from seven migraine studies. Cluster patients have just as much photophobia and phonophobia as migraine patients but less nausea and vomiting. Photophobia and phonophobia should not be considered good differentiating symptoms between cluster and migraine. Data derived from Rozen TD, Niknam RM, Shechter AL, *et al. J Neurol Neurosurg Psychiatr* 2001;70:613–7; Nappi G, Micieli G, Cavallini A, *et al. Cephalalgia* 1992;12:165–8; Vingen JV, Pareja JA, Sovner LJ. *Cephalalgia* 1998;18:250–6. n/a, data not available

| *Symptom* | *Rozen, 2001* | *Nappi, 1992 (n = seven studies)* | *Vingen, 1998* | *Migraine* |
|---|---|---|---|---|
| Photophobia | 80% | 56% | 91% | 79% |
| Phonophobia | 50% | 15% | 89% | 80% |
| Nausea | 53% | 41% | n/a | 87% |
| Vomiting | 32% | 24% | n/a | 56% |

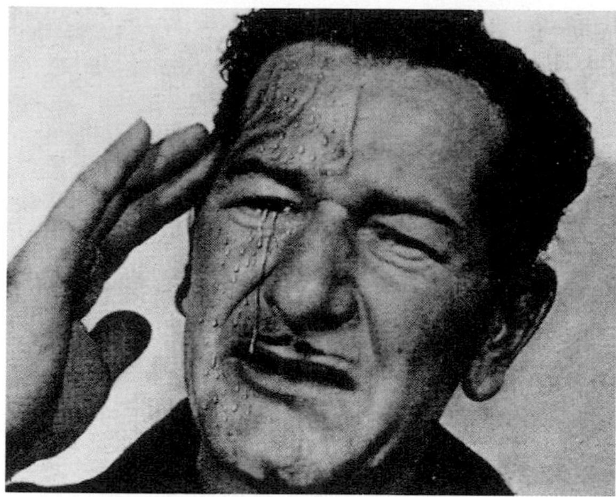

**Figure 6.11** An actual cluster patient of Bayard T. Horton. Horton is considered the 'father of cluster headache'; not only did he describe the cardinal features of cluster headache but he was also the first to use oxygen in its therapy. The image shows a male undergoing a right-sided cluster headache with associated autonomic symptoms. The patient has some of the typical 'leonine facies' features recognized in cluster headache: deep nasolabial folds, peau d'orange skin and squared jaw. Reproduced with permission from Horton BT. The use of histamine in the treatment of specific types of headaches. *JAMA* 1941;116:377–83

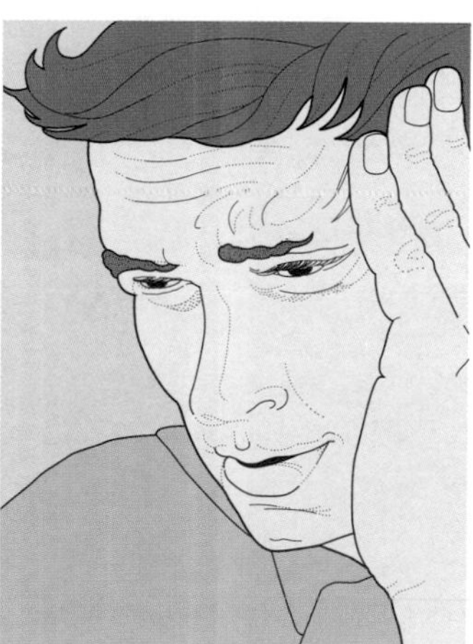

- Prevalence
- Predominantly male (male: female ratio)
- Rare before the age of ten years

**Figure 6.12** Cluster predominantly occurs in men, although more women are being diagnosed with cluster headache. The prevalence of cluster headache is 0.4% of the population. Adapted from the Neurology Ambassador Program with permission from the American Headache Society

frequently in cluster headaches as they do in migraine. Nausea and vomiting also occur in cluster patients, specifically females, but not nearly as frequently as in migraine (Table 6.5). With regard to the autonomic symptoms, which are hallmarks of cluster attacks (Figure 6.11), only about 50% of migraineurs have associated ptosis, unilateral lacrimation or nasal congestion/rhinorrhea with their headaches. In addition, aura, which was supposed to be a migraine-only event, has now been shown to occur with cluster headaches, so the presence of aura cannot define a primary headache syndrome. Finally, migraine is a disorder of women and cluster headache is supposed to be a disorder of men (Figure 6.12). It is not uncommon for physicians, falsely believing that women do not get cluster headaches, to give a woman a diagnosis of migraine just because she is a woman, even though she has typical cluster features. Cluster headaches undoubtedly occur in women, and a recent epidemiologic study from Italy suggests that more women are developing or being diagnosed with cluster headaches (Table 6.6). The

**Table 6.6** Data illustrating how the male:female cluster headache gender ratio is decreasing over time. The cause of this is unknown but may reflect a true increase in cluster incidence or better diagnoses by physicians. In total, 482 patients (374 males, 108 females) were evaluated. Reproduced with permission from reference 4

| *Male to female ratios* | |
|---|---|
| Before 1960 | 6.2:1 |
| 1960–1969 | 5.6:1 |
| 1970–1979 | 4.3:1 |
| 1980–1989 | 3.0:1 |
| 1990–1995 | 2.1:1 |

Is this due to a decrease in male cluster patients or an increase in females, or better diagnosis?

**Table 6.7** Abortive treatment of cluster headache. Sumatriptan injectable can provide relief within 5 min (Figure 6.13, Table 6.9). Oxygen is safe in all cluster patients, even those with cardiovascular risk factors (see also Table 6.8). Reproduced with permission from reference 1

| *High efficacy* |
|---|
| $O_2$ |
| sumatriptan subcutaneous (6 mg) |
| IV/IM/SQ dihydroergotamine mesylate 0.5–1.0 mg |
| *Limited efficacy* |
| zolmitriptan 5–10 mg oral |
| ergotamine 1–2 mg oral or suppository |
| intranasal lidocaine |

**Table 6.8** Oxygen is effective in up to 70% of cluster patients. A non-rebreather face mask should be used as delivery system. Reproduced with permission from reference 1

| |
|---|
| 100% $O_2$ 7–10 liters/min for 15 min |
| Efficacy 70% at 15 min |
| Most effective when headache is at maximum intensity |
| May delay rather than completely abort attack |
| Main limitation is accessibility |

**Table 6.9** Sumatriptan injectable is the fastest and most effective therapy for cluster headache at the present time. It is contraindicated in cluster patients with cardiovascular risk factors. Reproduced with permission from reference 1

| |
|---|
| Effective in 90% of patients for 90% of their attacks for both episodic and chronic cluster headache |
| Efficacy within 15 min in 50–75% |
| No tachyphylaxis |
| Not effective for cluster prophylaxis |

**Table 6.10** Surgical procedures for cluster headache are directed towards the sensory trigeminal nerve or cranial parasympathetic system (Figure 6.14). Surgery should only be considered once a patient is deemed refractory to medical treatment. Cluster patients who have only had one side of the head affected can get surgery in contrast to those who have had side-switching, as the latter are at great risk of having the headache switch sides after surgery

| |
|---|
| *Procedures directed towards the sensory trigeminal nerve* |
| Alcohol injection into supraorbital and infraorbital nerves |
| Alcohol injection into Gasserian ganglion |
| Avulsion of infraorbital/supraorbital/supratrochlear nerves |
| Retrogasserian glycerol injection (less corneal anesthesia) |
| Radiofrequency trigeminal gangliorhyzolysis (75% effective, 20% recurrence) |
| Trigeminal root section |
| *Procedures directed at autonomic pathways* |
| Section of greater superficial petrosal nerve |
| Section of nervus intermedius |
| *Neuromodulation* |
| Deep-brain stimulation of the ipsilateral posterior hypothalamus (Figure 6.24) |
| Greater occipital nerve stimulation |

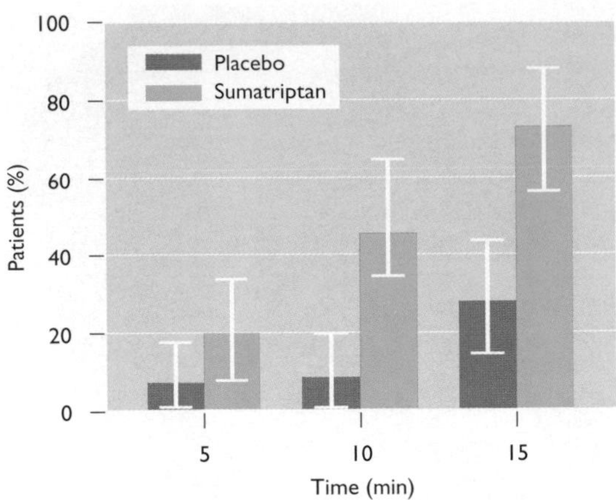


**Figure 6.13** Reduction in pain severity after administration of sumatriptan injectable to patients with cluster headache. A significant response was observed by 10 and 15 min versus placebo. Adapted with permission from Olesen J, Tfelt-Hansen P, Welch KMA, eds. *The Headaches*, 2nd edn. Philadelphia, PA: Lippincott Williams & Wilkins, 2000:733

- Sensory trigeminal pathway procedures
  - Radiofrequency or glycerol rhizotomy
  - Gamma knife radiosurgery
  - Trigeminal root section
  - Other
- Autonomic (parasympathetic) pathway procedures

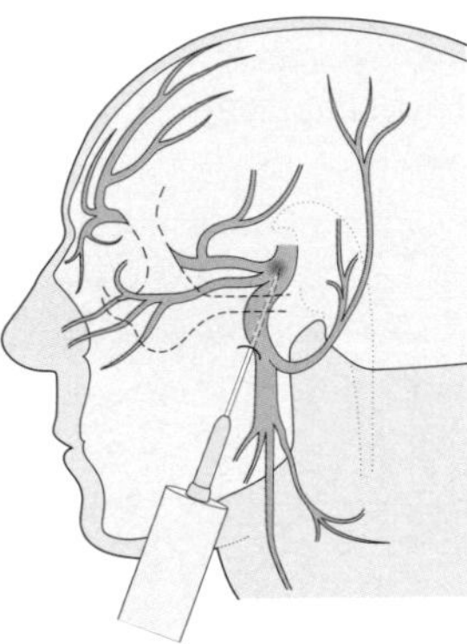

**Figure 6.14** Presently the most effective surgical therapy for cluster is radiofrequency lesioning of the gasserian (trigeminal) ganglion. Under radiographic control a device is inserted into the cheek and directed through the foramen ovale into the area of the gasserian ganglion where a specific denervating agent (radiofrequency, glycerol) is then used. Adapted from the Neurology Ambassador Program with permission from the American Headache Society

previous male:female cluster ratio of 6–7:1 decreased to 2:1 in the 1990s. Female cluster headaches can appear exactly like male cluster headaches except that female cluster patients develop more nausea and vomiting with cluster attacks and have less miosis and ptosis than their male counterparts.

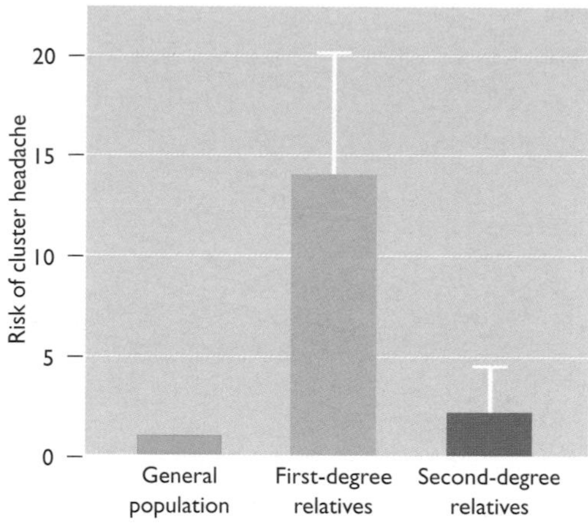


**Figure 6.15** Cluster is not considered to have a genetic predisposition as is seen in migraine, but first-degree relatives have a 14-fold increased risk of developing cluster headaches in their lifetime. Adapted with permission from Olesen J, Tfelt-Hansen P, Welch KMA, eds. *The Headaches*, 2nd edn. Philadelphia, PA: Lippincott Williams & Wilkins, 2000:680

- High alcohol/ tobacco usage
- Leonine facies (heavy facial features)
- Peau d'orange skin
- Hazel-colored eyes
- Duodenal ulceration
- Type A personality

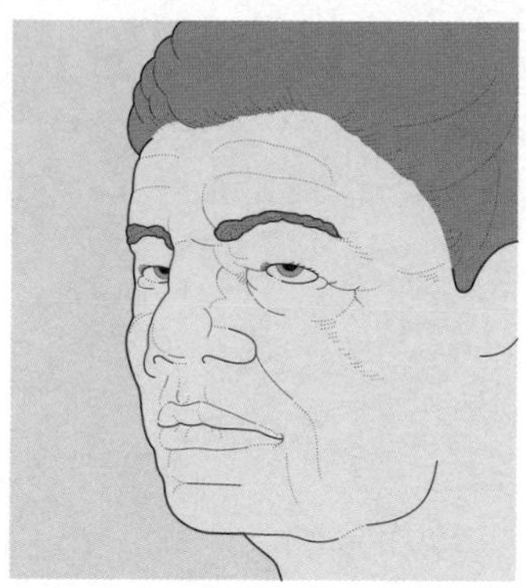

**Figure 6.16** Cluster headache has been linked to a typical facies, eye color and certain medical conditions. Adapted from the Neurology Ambassador Program with permission from the American Headache Society

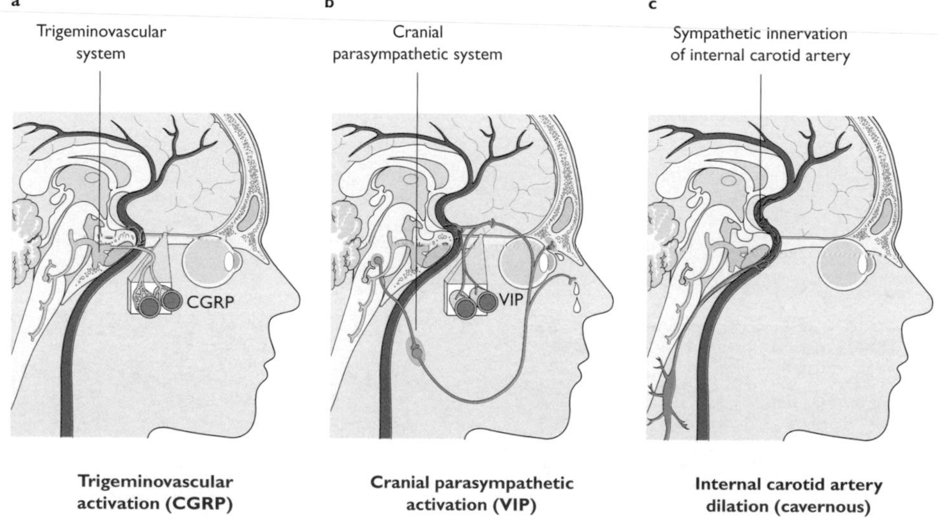


**Figure 6.17** The true pathogenesis of cluster headache is still unknown. What must be accounted for when determining a unified theory of cluster pathogenesis are: (a) The pain is orbital in location. This means the ipsilateral sensory trigeminal nerve system is involved. Trigeminal afferents transmit cephalic pain via the ophthalmic division of the trigeminal nerve synapse in the trigeminal ganglion which then relays this sensory input to the trigeminal nucleus caudalis in the brainstem. Calcitonin gene-related peptide (CGRP) is the neurotransmitter released in this system; (b) Ipsilateral symptoms of parasympathetic activation (lacrimation, nasal congestion). Cranial parasympathetic innervation of the intracranial vessels arise in primary order neurons in the superior salivatory nucleus in the pons. Efferents from this system (via the seventh cranial nerve) act to stimulate the nasal and lacrimal glands. Vasoactive intestinal peptide (VIP) is a marker of activation of the cranial parasympathetic system; (c) Ipsilateral symptoms of sympathetic dysfunction (miosis, ptosis, partial Horner's syndrome). As a result of activation of sensory trigeminal and cranial parasympathetic systems there is blood vessel dilation in the internal carotid artery. If the cavernous carotid artery (level at which the parasympathetic, sympathetic and trigeminal fibers converge) dilates, it can cause compression of the sympathetic system with the production of a post-ganglionic Horner's syndrome. Adapted from the Neurology Ambassador Program with permission from the American Headache Society

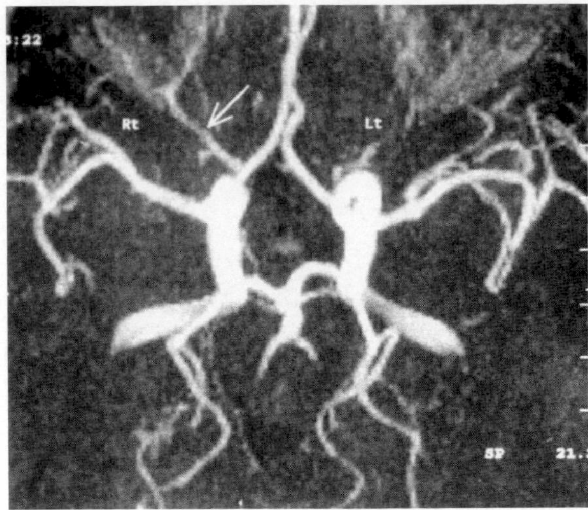


**Figure 6.18** Dilation of the ophthalmic artery during a spontaneous cluster attack. The artery normalized after cluster remission. Artery dilation in cluster headache may result from trigeminal nerve activation with release of calcitonin gene-related peptide (CGRP) or from an inflammatory process in the cavernous sinus and tributary veins leading to venous stasis and resultant artery dilation. Vascular congestion within the cavernous sinus region can explain the pain of cluster and the sympathetic damage seen during attacks. A venous vasculitis theory for cluster is another possible etiology for cluster pathogenesis. Reproduced with permission from Waldenlind E, Ekbom K, Torhall J. MR-angiography during spontaneous attacks of cluster headache: a case report. *Headache* 1993;33:291–5

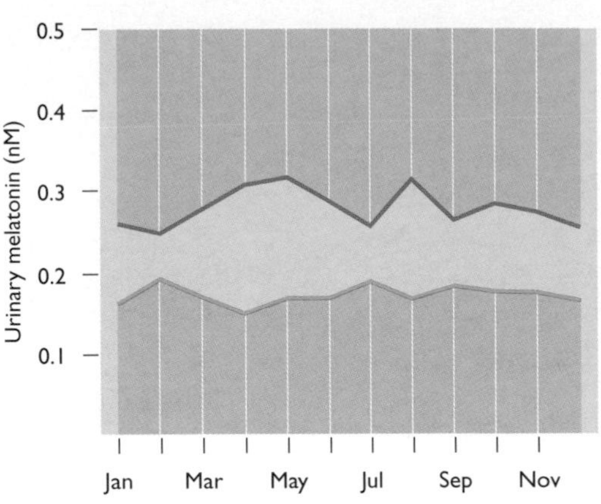


**Figure 6.19** Urine melatonin levels were examined for up to 14 months in episodic cluster headache patients (blue line) and healthy controls (purple line). The mean levels of urinary melatonin were significantly lower in patients than controls in both cluster periods and during remissions. Adapted from Waldenlind E, Gustafsson SA, Ekbom K, Wetterberg L. Circadian secretion of cortisol and melatonin in cluster headache during active cluster periods and remission. *J Neurol Neurosurg Psychiatr* 1987;50:207–13, with permission by the BMJ Publishing Group

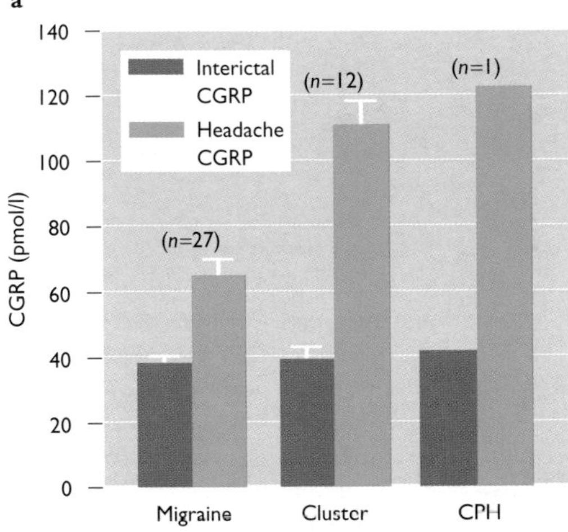


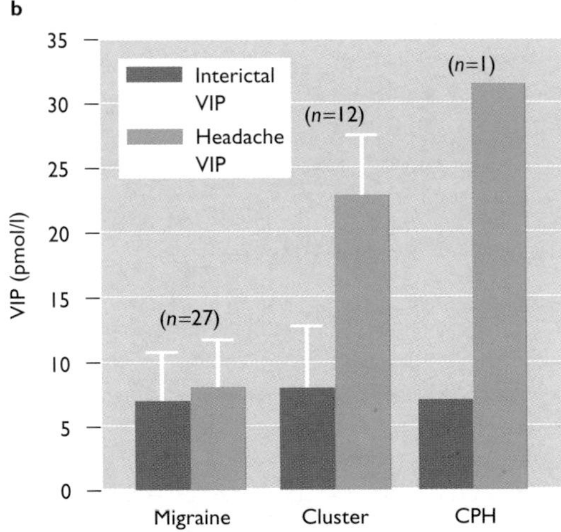


**Figure 6.20** Changes in calcitonin gene-related peptide (CGRP; a) and vasoactive intestinal polypeptide (VIP; b) levels during migraine, cluster and chronic paroxysmal hemicrania (CPH) attacks. Note elevation of both CGRP and VIP levels in the trigeminal-autonomic cephalgia (TAC) headaches but not in migraine. Adapted from Goadsby PJ, Lipton RB. A review of paroxysmal hemicranias, SUNCT syndrome and other short-lasting headaches with autonomic feature, including new cases. *Brain* 1997;120:193–209, with permission by Oxford University Press

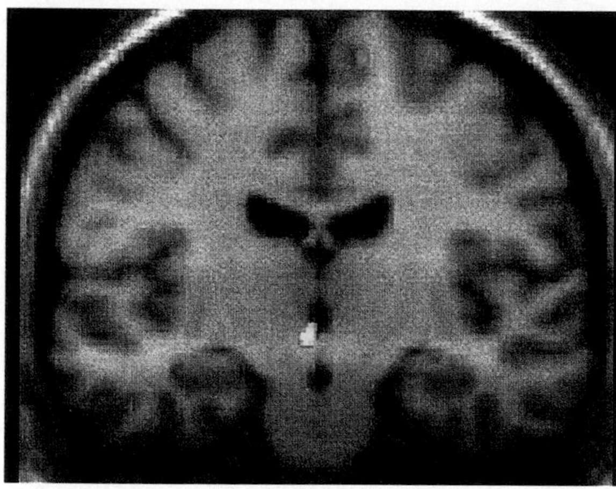

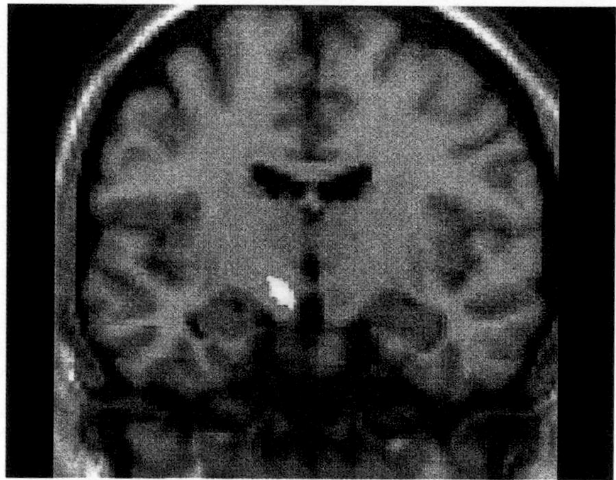

**Figure 6.21** Image on the left demonstrates hypothalamic activation during a cluster attack on PET. The image on the right is a voxel-based morphometric analysis of the structural T1-weighted MRI scans from 25 right-handed cluster patients revealing a significant difference in hypothalamic gray matter density (yellow) compared with non-cluster patients. The hypothalamus of cluster patients appears to have an increased volume compared with controls. Adapted from the Neurology Ambassador Program with permission from the American Headache Society

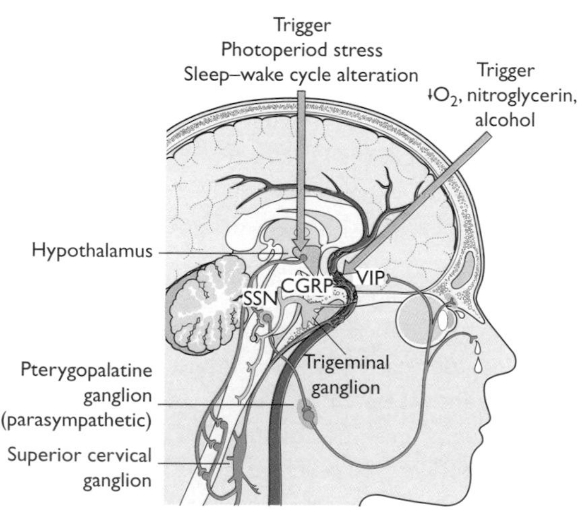


**Figure 6.22** Image showing how the hypothalamus, trigeminal sensory, cranial parasympathetic and carotid sympathetic systems interact to produce a cluster headache. The brainstem connection between the trigeminal and cranial sympathetic systems (trigeminal-autonomic reflex pathway) helps to explain the clinical phenotype of the trigeminal-autonomic cephalgias (TACs). CGRP, calcitonin gene-related peptide; SSN, superior salivatory nucleus; VIP, vasoactive intestinal polypeptide. Adapted from the Neurology Ambassador Program with permission from the American Headache Society

- Episodic → Chronic (13%)
- Chronic → Episodic (33%)
- Cluster-free intervals: 1.1 years → 3.5 years

**Figure 6.23** The natural history of cluster headaches is not well documented in the literature. About 13% of episodic cluster patients will develop into chronic cluster, whereas one-third of chronic cluster patients will change to episodic cluster. Being on a preventive appears to help with the latter transition. Most cluster patients will continue over their lifetime to have the same number of attacks per day and the same duration for each attack. Adapted from the Neurology Ambassador Program with permission from the American Headache Society

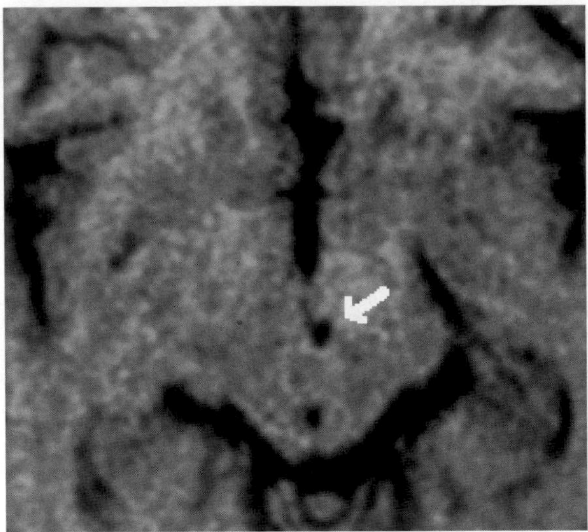

**Figure 6.24** Deep-brain hypothalamic stimulation for cluster headache. Axial T1-weighted post-operative magnetic resonance image showing the electrode (white arrow) within the posterior inferior left hypothalamus

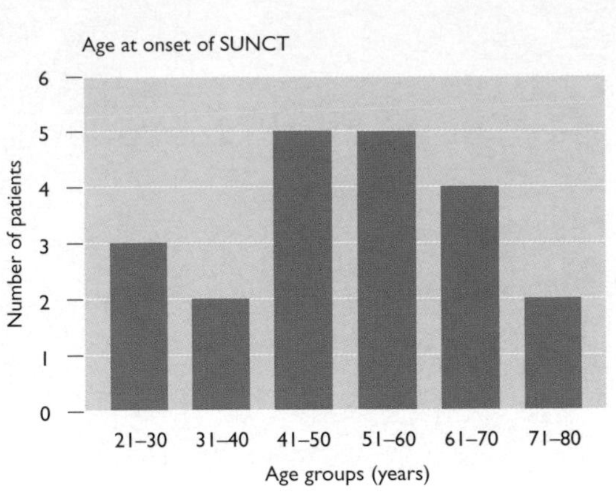


**Figure 6.25** SUNCT is considered a disorder of the elderly, although there are some reported cases younger than age 40. Adapted with permission from Pareja JA, Sjaastad O. SUNCT syndrome. A clinical review. *Headache* 1997;37:195–202

**Table 6.11** International Headache Society's criteria for SUNCT syndrome. Reproduced from reference 3, with permission of Blackwell Publishing

Diagnostic criteria:

A. At least 20 attacks fulfilling criteria B–D

B. Attacks of unilateral orbital, supraorbital or temporal stabbing or pulsating pain lasting 5–240 s

C. Pain is accompanied by ipsilateral conjunctival injection and lacrimation

D. Attacks occur with a frequency from 3 to 200 per day

E. Not attributed to another disorder[1]

Note:

1. History and physical and neurological examinations do not suggest any of the disorders listed in groups 5–12, or history and/or physical and/or neurological examinations do suggest such disorder but it is ruled out by appropriate investigations, or such disorder is present but attacks do not occur for the first time in close temporal relation to the disorder

## SUNCT

The syndrome of short-lasting unilateral neuralgiform headache attacks with conjunctival injection and tearing, or SUNCT, was first described by Sjaastad *et al.* in 1978 in an article entitled 'Multiple neuralgiform unilateral headache attacks associated with conjunctival injection and appearing in clusters'. The description of the complete syndrome came in 1989[5]. SUNCT is the rarest of the primary headache disorders. Many headache specialists have stated that they have never seen SUNCT. SUNCT comprises brief attacks of moderate to severe head pain with associated autonomic disturbances of conjunctival injection, tearing, rhinorrhea or nasal obstruction (Table 6.11). The typical age of onset is between 40 and 70 years (Figure 6.25). SUNCT pain is normally localized to an orbital or periorbital distribution, although the forehead and temple can be the main site of pain (Figure 6.26). Head pain can radiate to the temple, nose, cheek, ear and palate. The pain is normally side-locked and remains unilateral throughout an entire attack. In rare instances SUNCT pain can be bilateral. Pain severity is normally moderate to severe, unlike cluster headache pain which is always severe. The pain is described most often as a stabbing, burning, pricking or electric shock-like sensation. Pain duration is extremely short, lasting between 5 and 240 s, with an average duration of 10 to 60 s (Figure 6.1). It is this extremely brief pain duration that sets SUNCT apart from other primary headache syndromes; SUNCT pain normally plateaus at a maximum intensity for several seconds and then quickly abates. SUNCT can occur at any time of the day, and does not show a tendency towards nocturnal attacks; only 1.2% of reported sufferers have night-time episodes (Figure 6.27). Attack frequency varies greatly between

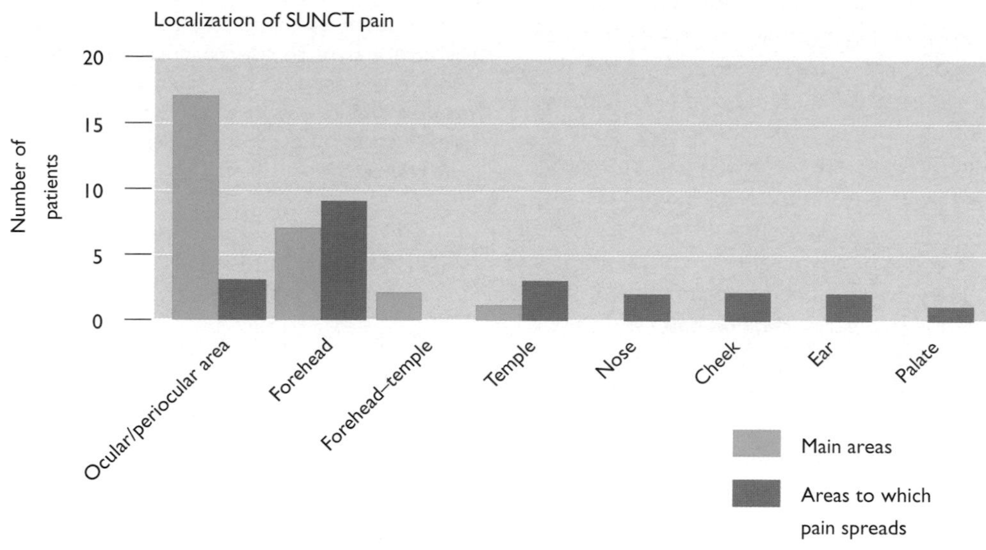


**Figure 6.26** SUNCT pain is located in or around the eye and/or the forehead region. It can spread to extra-trigeminal innervated areas. Adapted with permission from Pareja JA, Sjaastad O. SUNCT syndrome. A clinical review. *Headache* 1997;37:195–202

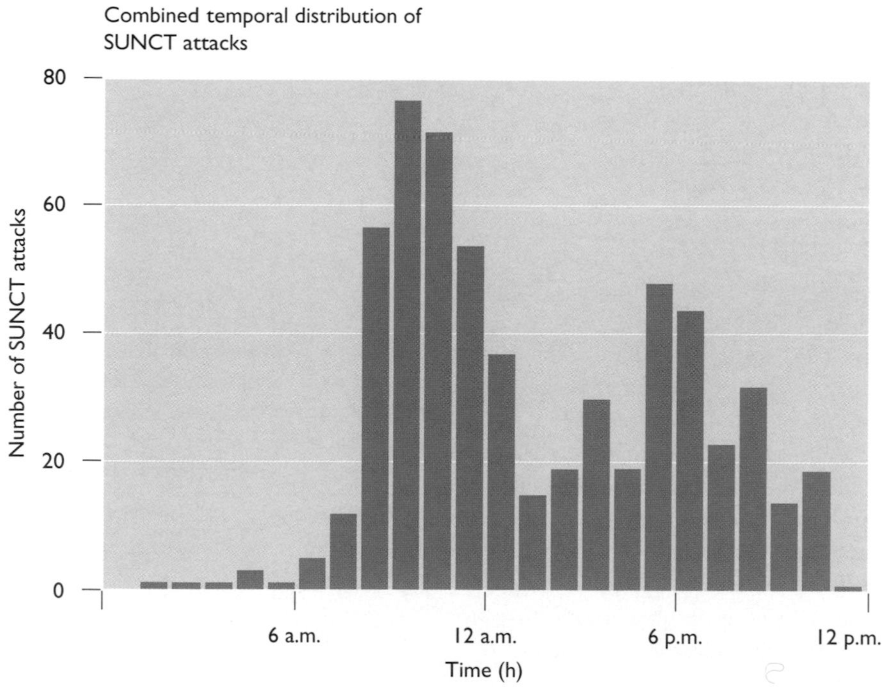


**Figure 6.27** SUNCT attacks tend to cluster around morning and afternoon/evening times, although attacks can occur at any time during the day. Adapted with permission from Pareja JA, Shen JM, Kruszewski P, *et al*. SUNCT syndrome: duration, frequency, and temporal distribution of attacks. *Headache* 1996;36:161–5

sufferers and within an individual sufferer. The usual attack frequency ranges anywhere from one to more than 80 episodes a day. Individuals can experience fewer than one attack an hour to more than 30. Mean attack frequency is 28 attacks per day. SUNCT is an episodic disorder that presents in a relapsing/remitting pattern. Each symptomatic period can last from several days to several months, and a person with SUNCT will typically have one to two symptomatic periods a year. The longest documented symptomatic period is five years, and the highest number of reported SUNCT episodes in one year is 22. Remissions typically last months but can last years. Symptomatic periods appear to increase in frequency and duration over time. All documented SUNCT patients experience conjunctival injection and lacrimation (ipsilateral to the side of the head pain) with each attack. Ipsilateral rhinorrhea and/or nasal obstruction occur in 67% of individuals. Less frequent associated symptoms include eyelid edema, a decreased palpebral fissure, facial redness, photophobia and blepharospasm (Table 6.12). Typically, conjunctival injection and eye tearing will start within 1–2 s of pain onset and remain until the head pain ceases, sometimes outlasting the pain by up to 30 s. Rhinorrhea, on the other hand, starts in the mid-to-late phase of an attack. Nausea, vomiting, photophobia and phonophobia are not normally associated with SUNCT. SUNCT can arise spontaneously, but many sufferers have identified triggering maneuvers, including mastication, nose blowing, coughing, forehead touching, eyelid squeezing, neck movements (rotation, extension and flexion) and ice cream eating. In SUNCT there is no refractory period between pain attacks, so that if a trigger zone is stimulated during the ending phase of a previous attack, a new one can begin immediately. This is unlike the refractory period of trigeminal neuralgia. The true epidemiology of SUNCT is not known, and there is no prevalence or incidence data available. The extremely low number of reported cases suggests it is a very rare syndrome. All patients with SUNCT must have an MRI to rule out secondary causes (Table 6.13). SUNCT does appear to have a clear male predominance, with a male:female ratio of 4.25:1[6]. SUNCT is typically a disease of middle-aged and older individuals. Up until recently there have been no reported therapies for SUNCT (Table 6.14), although several case reports documenting relief with lamotrigine, topiramate and gabapentin have come into the literature.

**Table 6.12** SUNCT attacks are marked by associated symptoms of parasympathetic activation (lacrimation, conjunctival injection) and much less common sympathetic dysfunction (ptosis); *symptomatic side; **symptomatic cases; †one patient reported bilateral nasal stenosis during attacks; ††reported as being bilateral by one patient. Reproduced with permission from reference 7

| | *n* |
|---|---|
| Lacrimation* | 21 (2**) |
| Conjunctival injection* | 20 (2**) |
| Rhinorrhea* | 14 (1**) |
| Nasal obstruction*† | 14 (1**) |
| Eyelid edema* | 8 (1**) |
| Decreased palpebral fissure* | 5 (1**) |
| Facial redness* | 4 (1**) |
| Tachypnea, clinically observable | 3 |
| Photophobia* | 2 |
| Blepharospasm†† | 2 |
| Miosis* | 1 |
| Feeling of facial sweating | 1 |
| Nausea | 1 |
| Ptosis | 1 |
| Feeling of foreign body in the eye* | 1 |
| Polyuria | 1 |
| Unpleasant feeling, nose | 1 |
| Dilated vessels, eyelids* | 1 |

**Table 6.13** All patients with SUNCT must have an MRI to rule out secondary causes, especially vascular malformation in the cerebellopontine region. MRI ($n$ = 12), CT ($n$ = 11), angiography ($n$ = 6); *symptomatic side, **symptomatic cases. Reproduced with permission from reference 7

| *Patient* | *Procedure* | *Results* |
|---|---|---|
| 2 | CT | Some enlarged sulci in frontal area |
| 3 | CT, MRI | Cholesteatoma* |
| 5<br>7 | MRI | Bilateral lacunar infarcts |
| 18 | Head X-ray | Osteoma in anterior part of scalp |
| 20**<br>21** | MRI, angiography | Vascular malformation in cerebellopontine region* |

**Table 6.14** Until recently multiple medications had been tried in SUNCT, all without success. Recently several case reports have documented the efficacy of lamotrigine, gabapentin and topiramate for SUNCT; –, treatment had no effect; x, treatment worsened condition; SC, subcutaneous; IV, intravenous; *one patient with slight improvement. Reproduced from reference 6, with permission of Oxford University Press

| *Treatment* | *Dosage (max/day)* | *Response* | *n* |
|---|---|---|---|
| *Pharmacologic* | | | |
| Aspirin | 1800 mg | – | 6 |
| Paracetamol | 4 g | – | 6 |
| Indomethacin | 200 mg | – | 9 |
| Naproxen | 1 g | – | 3 |
| Ibuprofen | 1200 mg | – | 3 |
| Ergotamine (oral) | 3 mg | – | 7 |
| Dihydroergotamine (IV) | 3 mg | – | 1 |
| Sumatriptan (oral) | 300 mg | –* | 5 |
| Sumatriptan (SC) | 6 mg | – | 1 |
| Prednisone (oral) | 100 mg | – | 7 |
| Methysergide | 8 mg | – | 4 |
| Verapamil | 480 mg | x | 5 |
| Valproate | 1500 mg | –* | 5 |
| Lithium | 900 mg | – | 3 |
| Propranolol | 160 mg | – | 3 |
| Amitriptyline | 100 mg | – | 2 |
| Carbamazepine | 1200 mg | – | 10 |
| *Procedures or infusions* | | | |
| Lignocaine (IV) | 4 mg/min | – | 2 |
| Greater occipital nerve block | | – | 4 |

## CHRONIC PAROXYSMAL HEMICRANIA

Chronic paroxysmal hemicrania is a very rare headache syndrome first described by Sjaastad and Dale in 1974[8] (Table 6.15). The new IHS criteria for chronic paroxysmal hemicrania are in Table 6.16. Unlike cluster headaches and SUNCT, CPH has a female predominance, with a female:male ratio of 3:1. CPH normally develops in the second or third decade of life but it can occur at any age (Figures 6.31 and 6.32). The natural history of this disorder is unknown (Figure 6.33). Clinically CPH patients have strictly unilateral headaches and the same side of the head is always affected. The pain location is normally orbital, temporal and above or behind the ear. The pain is very severe and is described as boring or claw-like (Figure 6.34). Attacks are short-lasting, between 2 and 30 min. Individuals can have between one and 40 attacks in a day; median frequency is five to ten attacks per day. Unlike cluster headache there is no predilection for nocturnal attacks, although CPH attacks can certainly awaken patients from sleep (Figure 6.35). Most CPH patients exhibit associated symptoms of lacrimation (62%), followed by nasal congestion (42%), conjunctival injection and rhinorrhea (36%) and ptosis (33%) (Table 6.17). Neck movements and external pressure to the transverse processes of C4 to C5 or the C2 nerve root can trigger CPH attacks. In phenotype, CPH is characterized by short-duration and more frequent cluster attacks. Unlike cluster patients, CPH patients typically remain still during an attack and by definition CPH responds to indomethacin treatment (Table 6.16). It does not matter how many years a patient has suffered from CPH and how many therapies they have tried, once indomethacin is administered the headaches will be gone within 48 h and remain alleviated as long as the patient remains on indomethacin (Figure 6.36). Very few other medications have ever worked for patients with CPH (Table 6.18). Secondary causes of CPH reported in the literature include: gangliocytoma of the sella turcica, pancoast tumor, frontal lobe tumor and cavernous sinus menigioma.

Episodic paroxysmal hemicrania (EPH) is characterized by frequent daily attacks of unilateral short-

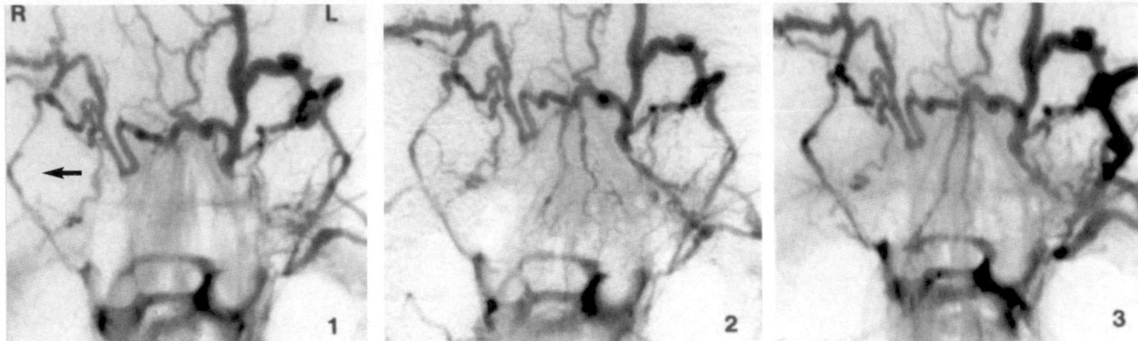


**Figure 6.28** Orbital phlebography in a 49-year-old man with SUNCT. On the side of the pain on the right (see arrow), there was narrowing of the whole superior ophthalmic vein (1 and 2). Orbital phlebography completed when the patient was in a remission state was normal (3). The findings suggest that SUNCT, at least in a subset of patients, may be caused by a venous vasculitis. Reproduced with permission from Hannerz J, Greitz D, Hansson P, Ericson K. SUNCT may be another manifestation of orbital venous vasculitis. *Headache* 1992;32:384–9

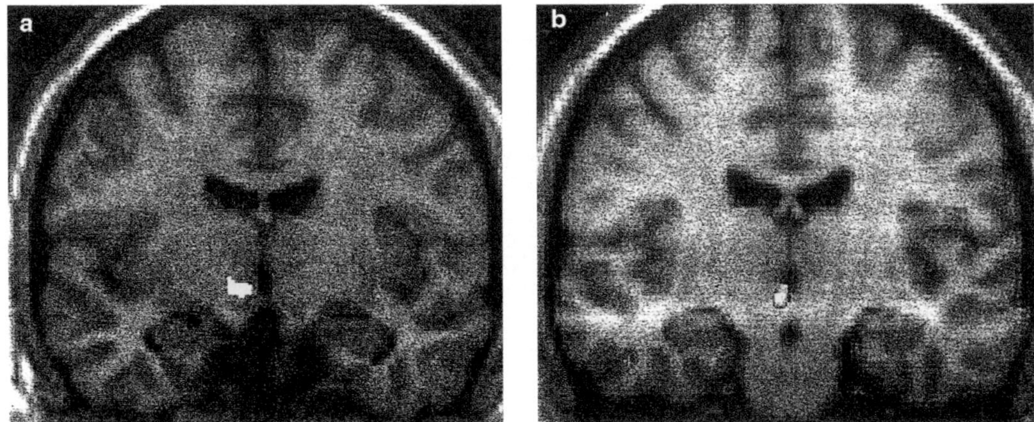


**Figure 6.29** BOLD contrast-MRI of the brain of a 71-year-old woman with SUNCT syndrome. (a) Activation is noted in the ipsilateral posterior hypothalamic gray region (yellow). Almost the same exact area of activation is noted during a cluster attack (b) suggesting a similar underlying cause of these clinically disparate TACs. Adapted with permission from May A, Bahra A, Buchel C, *et al*. Functional magnetic resonance imaging in spontaneous attacks of SUNCT: Short-lasting neuralgiform headache with conjunctival injection and tearing. *Ann Neurol* 1999;46:791–4, copyright John Wiley & Sons, Inc

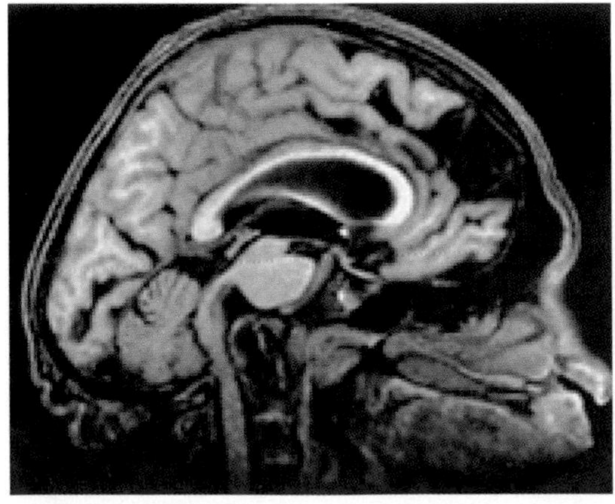

**Figure 6.30** Patient with history of osteogenesis imperfecta presented with short-lasting attacks of left sided sharp, excruciating pain with a duration of 2–3 min and a frequency of one to five times a day in association with nausea, ipsilateral lacrimation, facial flushing, conjunctival injection, and bilateral rhinorrhea. After some months the duration increased to 30–60 min, and the pain quality changed to a deep excruciating, boring pain with 10–15 episodes a day of superimposed lancinating pain. Midline sagittal T1 weighted MRI image of the cranium and craniocervical junction of the patient with osteogenesis imperfecta and possible symptomatic SUNCT. Severe platybasia with marked basilar impression and distortion of the posterior fossa anatomical relations. The odontoid process produces pronounced pontomedullary angulation. Reproduced with permission from Berg JWM, Goadsby PJ. Significance of atypical presentation of symptomatic SUNCT: a case report. *J Neurol Neurosurg Psychiatry* 2001;70:244–6

**Table 6.15** Chronic paroxysmal hemicrania (CPH) is a relatively rare condition even in headache specialty clinics. By 1989, 84 cases had been described in the literature. CPH case reports are no longer published because this syndrome is now recognized as a true primary headache disorder. Reproduced with permission from reference 9

| *Published case reports* | *Year* | *n* |
|---|---|---|
| Sjaastad & Dale | 1974 | 2 |
| Sjaastad & Dale | 1976 | 1 |
| Kayed *et al.* | 1978 | 1 |
| Price & Posner | 1978 | 1 |
| Christoffersen | 1979 | 1 |
| Manzoni & Terzano | 1979 | 1 |
| Leblanc *et al.* | 1980 | 1 |
| Sjaastad *et al.* | 1980 | 2 |
| Stein & Rogado | 1980 | 2 |
| Guerra | 1981 | 2 |
| Hochman | 1981 | 1 |
| Manzoni *et al.* | 1981 | 1 |
| Rapoport *et al.* | 1981 | 1 |
| Jensen *et al.* | 1982 | 1 |
| Kilpatrick & King | 1982 | 2 |
| Pelz & Meskey | 1982 | 1 |
| Geaney | 1983 | 1 |
| Peatty & Clifford Rose | 1983 | 1 |
| Thevenet *et al.* | 1983 | 3 |
| Bogucki *et al.* | 1984 | 2 |
| Boulliat | 1984 | 1 |
| Dutta | 1984 | 1 |
| Pfaffenrath *et al.* | 1984 | 4 |
| Pradalier & Dry | 1984 | 1 |
| Sjaastad *et al.* | 1984 | 2 |
| Drummond | 1985 | 1 |
| Granella *et al.* | 1985 | 3 |
| Heckl | 1986 | 2 |
| Pollman & Pfaffenrath | 1986 | 1 |
| Bogucki & Kozubski | 1987 | 1 |
| Centonze *et al.* | 1987 | 3 |
| Durko & Klimek | 1987 | 1 |
| Hannerz *et al.* | 1987 | 1 |
| Joubert *et al.* | 1987 | 1 |
| Kudrow *et al.* | 1987 | 6 |
| Nebudova | 1987 | 1 |
| Rasmussen | 1987 | 4 |
| Pearce *et al.* | 1987 | 1 |
| | Sum: | 63 |
| *Unpublished case reports* | | |
| Bousser | | 2 |
| Davalos | | 1 |
| Graham | | 1 |
| Greene | | 1 |
| Jaeger | | 2 |
| Manzoni | | 1 |
| Mathew | | 2 |
| Nappi | | 2 |
| Sjaastad | | 8 |
| Wall | | 1 |
| | Sum: | 21 |
| | Total: | 84 |

duration headaches with associated autonomic symptoms. EPH is really CPH, except EPH has periods of headache remission lasting weeks or months (Table 6.16 and Figure 6.33). There is debate if EPH is just an episodic variant of CPH or its own entity. Attack duration in EPH varies from 1 to

**Table 6.16** International Headache Society's criteria for chronic paroxysmal hemicrania and episodic paroxysmal hemicrania. Reproduced from reference 3, with permission of Blackwell Publishing

*Paroxysmal hemicrania*

Diagnostic criteria:

A. At least 20 attacks fulfilling criteria B–D
B. Attacks of severe unilateral orbital, supraorbital or temporal pain lasting 2–30 min
C. Headache is accompanied by at least one of the following:
   1. ipsilateral conjunctival injection and/or lacrimation
   2. ipsilateral nasal congestion and/or rhinorrhea
   3. ipsilateral eyelid edema
   4. ipsilateral forehead and facial sweating
   5. ipsilateral miosis and/or ptosis
D. Attacks have a frequency above five per day for more than half of the time, although periods with lower frequency may occur
E. Attacks are prevented completely by therapeutic doses of indomethacin[1]
F. Not attributed to another disorder[2]

Notes:

1. In order to rule out incomplete response, indomethacin should be used in a dose of $\geq$ 150 mg daily orally or rectally, or $\geq$ 100 mg by injection, but for maintenance smaller doses are often sufficient

2. History and physical and neurological examinations do not suggest any of the disorders listed in groups 5–12, or history and/or physical and/or neurological examinations do suggest such disorder but it is ruled out by appropriate investigations, or such disorder is present but attacks do not occur for the first time in close temporal relation to the disorder

*Episodic paroxysmal hemicrania*

Diagnostic criteria:

A. Attacks fulfilling criteria A–F for paroxysmal hemicrania
B. At least two attack periods lasting 7–365 days and separated by pain-free remission periods of $\geq$ 1 month

*Chronic paroxysmal hemicrania (CPH)*

Diagnostic criteria:

A. Attacks fulfilling criteria A–F for paroxysmal hemicrania
B. Attacks recur over $>$ 1 year without remission periods or with remission periods lasting $<$ 1 month

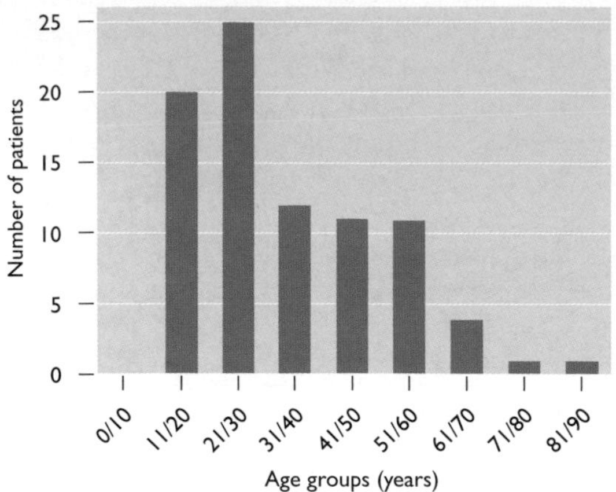


**Figure 6.31** Chronic paroxysmal hemicrania (CPH) typically starts to occur in the teens or twenties, very similar to the age of onset of cluster. Adapted with permission from Antonaci F, Sjaastad O. Chronic paroxysmal hemicrania (CPH): a review of the clinical manifestations. *Headache* 1989;29: 648–56

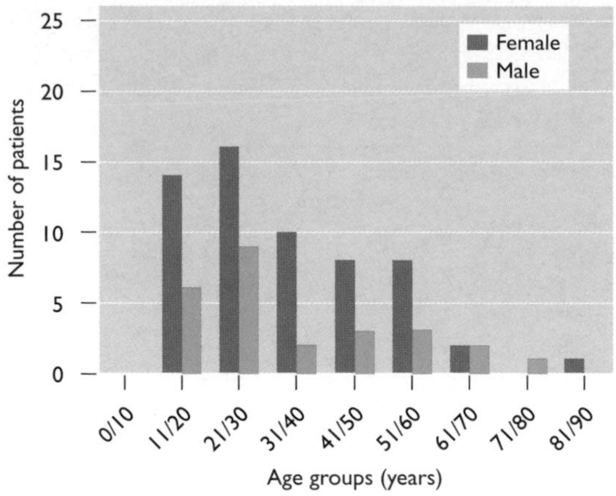

**Figure 6.32** Both females and males who develop chronic paroxysmal hemicrania (CPH) typically have their first attacks in their teens or twenties. Adapted with permission from Antonaci F, Sjaastad O. Chronic paroxysmal hemicrania (CPH): a review of the clinical manifestations. *Headache* 1989;29: 648–56

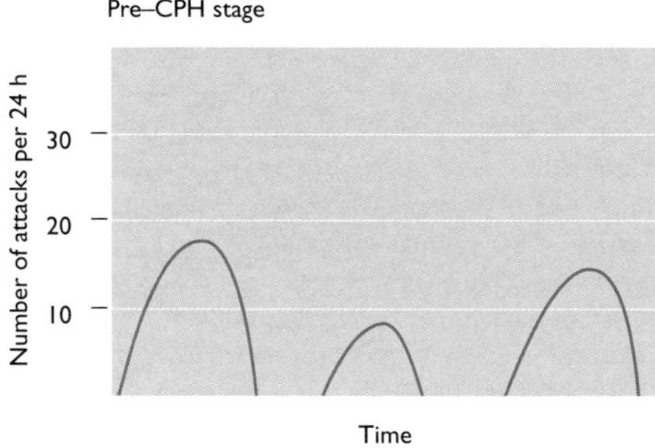


**Figure 6.33** The natural history of chronic paroxysmal hemicrania (CPH) is unknown. When Sjaastad first identified CPH he noticed that some patients went through a pre-CPH stage of CPH attacks with remission periods. In some patients these patients never went on to have CPH. Most likely this pre- CPH stage is episodic paroxysmal hemicrania (EPH). Adapted with permission from Russell D, Sjaastad O. Chronic paroxysmal hemicrania. In: Pfaffenrath V, Sjaastad O, Lundberg PO, eds. *Updating in Headache*. Berlin: Springer-Verlag, 1984:1–6, copyright Springer-Verlag

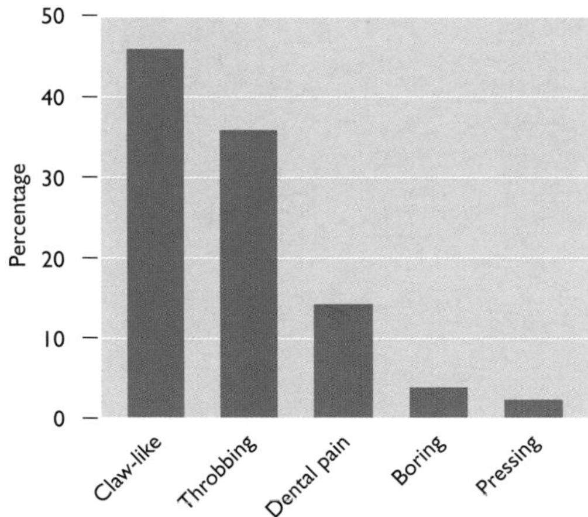


**Figure 6.34** Quality of chronic paroxysmal hemicrania (CPH) pain. Adapted with permission from Antonaci F, Sjaastad O. Chronic paroxysmal hemicrania (CPH): a review of the clinical manifestations. *Headache* 1989;29:648–56

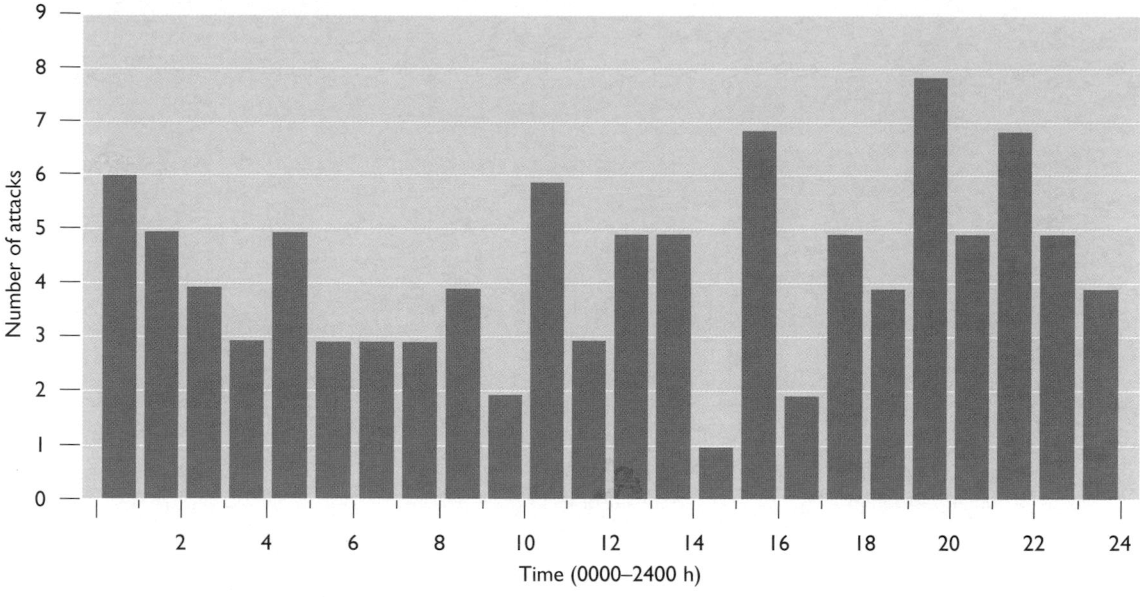


**Figure 6.35** Chronic paroxysmal hemicrania attacks, unlike cluster attacks, occur anytime during the day and night and do not have a predilection for nocturnal attacks. Adapted with permission from Russell D. Chronic paroxysmal hemicrania: severity, duration and time of occurrence of attacks. *Cephalalgia* 1984;4:53–6

**Table 6.17** Autonomic symptoms mark the chronic paroxysmal hemicrania syndrome, specifically those suggesting cranial parasympathetic activation. Reproduced with permission from reference 9

| *Symptoms and signs* | *n* |
|---|---|
| Lacrimation | 52 |
| Nasal stenosis | 35 |
| Conjunctival injection | 30 |
| Rhinorrhea | 30 |
| Ptosis | 28 |
| Photophobia | 18 |
| Miosis | 15 |
| Nausea | 12 |
| Generalized sweating | 8 |
| V1 hypersensitivity | 7 |
| Phonophobia | 6 |
| Temporal artery pulsation | 5 |
| Visual phenomena | 4 |
| Temporal artery dilatation | 4 |
| Tinnitus | 3 |
| Vomiting | 2 |
| $V_2$ hypersensitivity | 2 |
| Exophthalmus | 1 |

**Table 6.18** Chronic paroxysmal hemicrania (CPH) is one of the indomethacin-responsive headache syndromes. When a CPH patient cannot tolerate indomethacin or has contraindications to this drug, there are very few, if any other, medications that work in this disorder. Reproduced with permission from reference 9

| *Drug reports* | *Partial efficacy of reports* | *Total number* |
|---|---|---|
| Salicylates | 25 | 37 |
| Ergotamine | 3 | 36 |
| Prednisone | 2 | 18 |
| β-Receptor blocking agents | 0 | 13 |
| Pizotifen | 0 | 11 |
| Carbamazepine | 0 | 11 |
| Lithium | 1 | 11 |
| Amitriptyline | 0 | 8 |
| Ketoprofen | 1 | 7 |
| Methysergide | 0 | 7 |
| Butazolidin | 1 | 6 |
| Naproxen | 4 | 5 |
| Phenobarbital | 0 | 5 |
| Oxygen | 0 | 4 |
| Tiapride | 0 | 3 |
| Ibuprofen | 0 | 3 |
| Diclofenac | 2 | 2 |
| Valproate | 0 | 1 |
| Verapamil | 0 | 1 |
| Clonazepam | 0 | 1 |
| Nimodipine | 0 | 1 |
| Histamine | 0 | 1 |
| Placebo | 0 | 7 |

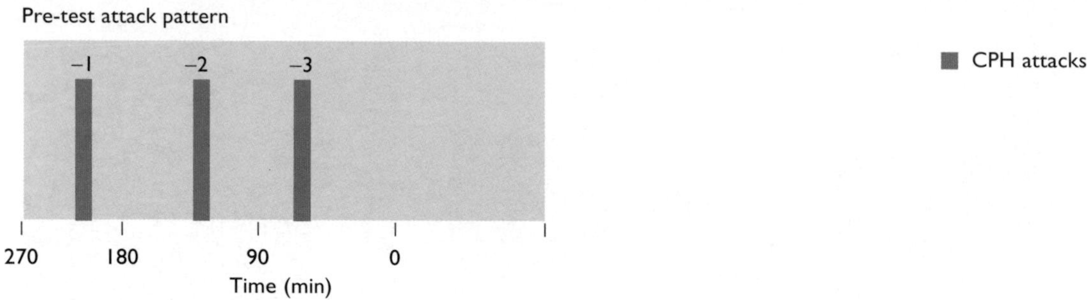


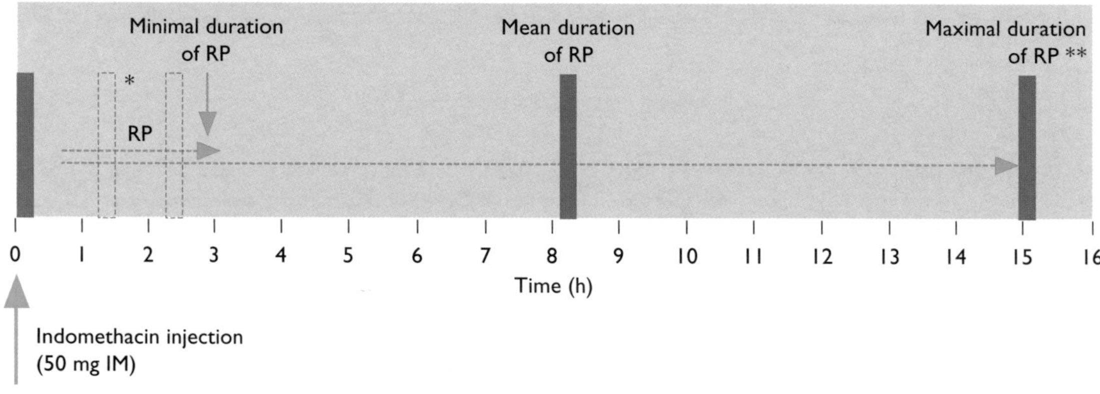


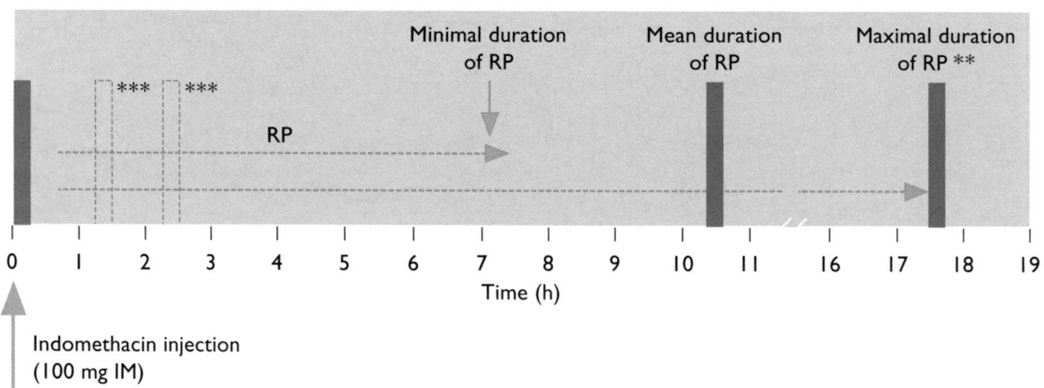


**Figure 6.36** Indomethacin is the sole treatment of choice in chronic paroxysmal hemicrania (CPH). Antonaci *et al.* have described the 'indotest' in which a 50 mg indomethacin IM test dosage can be given to patients in the office with possible CPH. When looking at the mean interval of attack frequency pre-indomethacin and post-indomethacin, after indomethacin the attack frequency is reduced (refractory period (RP) was initiated post-indomethacin). If a patient after indomethacin does not get their typical next attack, then indomethacin should be effective in that patient for their headaches. *Hatched lines indicate putative attacks that have not materialized; **pre-attack pattern re-established in all patients; ***the timing of the anticipated attacks is not based on exact recording of the attack pattern prior to the 100 mg test. Adapted with permission from Antonaci F, Pareja JA, Caminero AB, Sjaastad O. Chronic paroxysmal hemicrania and hemicrania continua. Parenteral indomethacin: the 'indotest'. *Headache* 1998;38:122–8

30 min, with attack frequency between 6 and 30 individual headaches per day. EPH, unlike CPH, may not have a gender predominance. EPH, like CPH, invariably responds to indomethacin. There are reports in the literature of transformation from EPH to CPH suggesting these two conditions are ends of a spectrum.

## REFERENCES


1. American Headache Society. Neurology Ambassador Program. http://www.ahsnet.org/ambass/ 3/27/2002
2. Klapper JA, Klapper A, Voss T. The misdiagnosis of cluster headache: a nonclinic, population-based Internet survey. *Headache* 2000;40:730–5
3. Headache Classification Subcommittee of the International Headache Society. The International Classification of Headache Disorders, 2nd Edn. *Cephalalgia* 2004;24(Suppl 1):1–150
4. Manzoni GC. Male preponderance of cluster headache progressively decreasing over the years. *Headache* 1997;35:588–9
5. Sjaastad O, Saunte C, Salvesen R, *et al.* Shortlasting unilateral neuralgiform headache attacks with conjunctival injection, tearing, sweating, and rhinorrhea. *Cephalalgia* 1989;9:147–56
6. Goadsby PJ, Lipton RB. A review of paroxysmal hemicranias, SUNCT syndrome and other short-lasting headaches with automatic feature, including new cases. *Brain* 1997;120:193–209
7. Pareja JA, Sjaastad O. SUNCT syndrome. A clinical review. *Headache* 1997;37:195–202
8. Sjaastad O, Dale I. Evidence for a new, treatable headache entity. *Headache* 1997;14:105–8
9. Antonaci F, Sjaastad O. Chronic paroxysmal hemicrania (CPH): a review of the clinical manifestations. *Headache* 1989;29:648–56

# 7

# Tension-type headaches

William B Young

## INTRODUCTION

The most controversial and difficult boundary among primary headaches is the one between migraine and tension-type headache. While some view these disorders as distinct entities, others favor the 'spectrum' or 'continuum' concept, the idea that migraine and tension-type headache exist as polar ends on a continuum of severity, varying more in degree than in kind (Figure 7.1). Lipton *et al.*[1] in the 'spectrum' study found that migrainous and tension-type headaches in migraine patients responded to sumatriptan, supporting the spectrum theory. In the early phase of a migraine headache, the patient may have mild, non-pulsating pain and a lack of nausea, vomiting, photophobia and phonophobia, in which case the headache resembles a tension-type headache. Individuals often report only the symptoms of tension-type headache, yet have headaches that respond to migraine-specific treatment on prospective diary studies.

The International Headache Society (IHS)[2] classification of headache, published in 2004, defined diagnostic criteria for primary headaches, including migraine and tension-type headaches (see Table 7.1). These criteria were more complete, explicit, and rigorous than criteria used in past studies, and led to an important advance in the research of headache disorders. However, tension-type headache was defined as recurrent headache without the features of migraine, perhaps artificially dividing a single disorder.

## EPIDEMIOLOGY

Tension-type headache is the most common headache type. Estimates of its prevalence have varied widely. In Western countries, 1-year prevalence ranges from 28–63% in men and from 34–86% in women, depending, in part, on methodologic differences between studies. A lifetime preva-

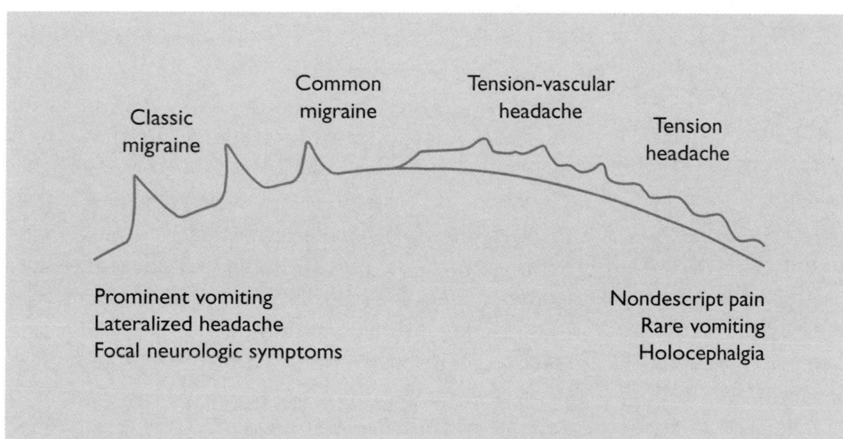


**Figure 7.1** 'The continuum of benign recurring headache' was introduced by Raskin. Adapted with permission from Raskin NH. *Headache*, 2nd edn. New York: Churchill Livingstone, 1988:215–24

lence of 69% in men and 88% in women, and a 1-year prevalence of 63% in men and 86% in women, was found in Denmark[3]. Interestingly, in mainland China there was a very low prevalence of tension-type headache[4].

The prevalence of chronic tension-type headache has varied from 2–3% in three Western studies[3,5].

## PATHOPHYSIOLOGY

The term tension-type headache represents a compromise between those who believed this entity to be due to psychologic tension and those who felt muscle tension to be paramount. Ultimately, very little is known about the pathophysiology of tension-type headache. The IHS recognizes tension-type headache with and without a pericranial muscle disorder. Muscle tenderness may be seen in migraine, and findings in EMG and pressure algometry studies are inconsistent, even in the pericranial muscle abnormality group of tension-type headache patients.

## IMPACT AND COSTS

Tension-type headaches often interfere with activities of daily living[6]. Eighteen percent of tension-type headache sufferers had to discontinue normal activity, while 44% experienced some limitation of function. Like migraine, tension-type headache is a disorder of middle life, striking individuals early in life and continuing to affect them through their peak productive years. All migraineurs, and 60% of tension-type headache patients, have a diminished capacity for work or other activities during an attack. In a Danish study, 43% of employed migraineurs and 12% of employed tension-type headache sufferers missed one or more days of work because of headache. Migraine caused at least one day of missed work for 5% of sufferers, while tension-type headache caused a day of missed work for 9%. Annually, per 1000 employed individuals, 270 lost work days were due to migraine and 820 were due to tension-type headache. Despite prominent disability, nearly 50% of migraineurs and more than 80% of tension-type headache patients had never consulted their general practitioner because of headache[7]. Patients with daily headaches may have even more disability than episodic migraine and tension-type headache sufferers, although there are no data to confirm this assumption.

**Table 7.1** IHS criteria for migraine and tension-type headache

*Migraine*

A. At least five attacks fulfilling criteria B–D
B. Headache attacks lasting 4–72 h (untreated or unsuccessfully treated)
C. Headache has at least two of the following characteristics:
   1. unilateral location
   2. pulsating quality
   3. moderate or severe pain intensity
   4. aggravation by or causing avoidance of routine physical activity(e.g. walking or climbing stairs)
D. During headache at least one of the following:
   1. nausea and/ or vomiting
   2. photophobia and phonophobia
E. Not attributed to another disorder

*Tension-type headache*

A. At least ten episodes fulfilling criteria B–D
B. Headache lasting 30 min to 7 days
C. Headache has at least two of the following characteristics:
   1. bilateral location
   2. pressing/ tightening (non-pulsatile) quality
   3. mild or moderate intensity
   4. not aggravated by routine physical activity such as walking or climbing stairs
D. Both of the following:
   1. no nausea or vomiting (anorexia may occur)
   2. no more than one of photophobia or phonophobia
E. Not attributed to another disorder

Adapted with permission from reference 2

## CONCLUSIONS

The pathophysiology of tension-type headache is not clearly understood. Raskin introduced the headache 'continuum' in 1988. In the last decade the pathogenesis of tension-type headache has again been called into question (Figure 7.2). Patients with migraine often suffer from milder headaches which meet the IHS criteria for tension-type headache[8,9]. These milder tension-type headaches seen in migraineurs often have a few associated migrainous features such as phonophobia or photophobia[10]. Cady *et al.*[11] observed that non-IHS migraine and tension-type headaches in patients with migraine respond to triptans, supporting theories of a common pathophysiology. Lipton *et al.*[1] demonstrated that in patients with migraine, sumatriptan was effective for

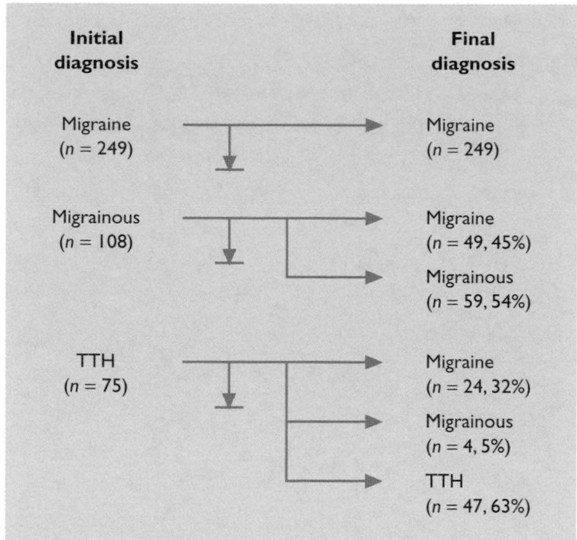


**Figure 7.2** Reclassification of headache diagnosis based on diary review. TTH, tension-type headache. Adapted from Lipton RB, Stewart WF, Hall C, et al. The misdiagnosis of disabling episodic headache: Results from the Spectrum Study. Presented at the International Headache Congress, June 2001

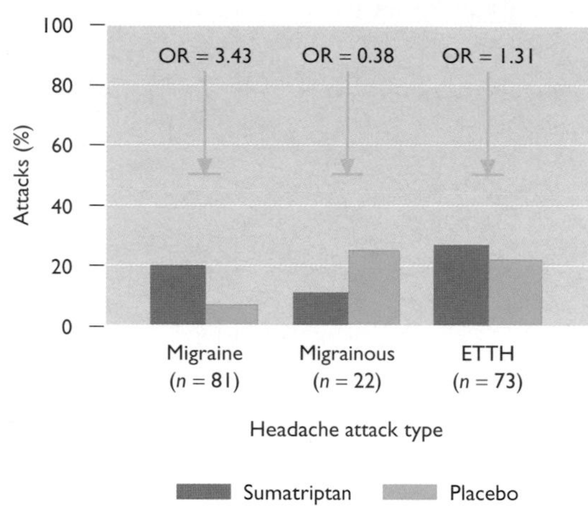


**Figure 7.3** Pain-free response at 2 h by headache attack type in individuals with an initial diagnosis of tension-type headache and a final diagnosis of migraine. ETTH, episodic tension-type headache; OR, odds ratio. Adapted with kind permission of Richard B. Lipton

their tension-type headaches (Figure 7.3). Tension-type headaches in patients with no migraine history seemingly lack migrainous features and do not respond to triptans[12,13]. To clarify these issues a prospective trial is needed testing triptans in migraineurs and non-migraineurs[14].

## REFERENCES

1. Lipton RB, Stewart WF, Cady R, *et al.* 2000 Wolff Award. Sumatriptan for the range of headaches in migraine sufferers: results of the Spectrum Study. *Headache* 2000;40:783–91
2. Headache Classification Subcommittee of the International Headache Society. The International Classification of Headache Disorders, 2nd edn. *Cephalalgia* 2004;24[Suppl 1]:1–150
3. Rasmussen BK, Jensen R, Schroll M, Olesen J. Epidemiology of headache in a general population – a prevalence study. *J Clin Epidemiol* 1991;44: 1147–57
4. Wong TW, Wong KS, Yu TS, Kay R. Prevalence of migraine and other headaches in Hong Kong. *Neuroepidemiology* 1995;14:82–91
5. Castillo J, Munoz P, Guitera V, *et al.* Epidemiology of chronic daily headache in the general population. *Headache* 1999;39:190–6
6. Rasmussen BK. Epidemiology and socio-economic impact of headache. *Cephalalgia* 1999;19:20–3
7. Rasmussen BK, Olesen J. Symptomatic and nonsymptomatic headaches in a general population. *Neurology* 1992;42:1225–31
8. Rasmussen BK, Jensen R, Schroll M, Olesen J. Interrelations between migraine and tension-type headache in the general population. *Arch Neurol* 1992;49:914–18
9. Ulrich V, Russell MB, Jensen R, Olesen J. A comparison of tension-type headache in migraineurs and in non-migraineurs: a population-based study. *Pain* 1996;67:501–6
10. Iversen HK, Langemark M, Andersson PG, *et al.* Clinical characteristics of migraine and episodic tension-type headache in relation to old and new diagnostic criteria. *Headache* 1990;30:514–19
11. Cady RK, Gutterman D, Saiers JA, Beach ME. Responsiveness of non-IHS migraine and tension-type headache to sumatriptan. *Cephalalgia* 1997;17: 588–90

12. Brennum J, Kjeldsen M, Olesen J. The 5-$HT_1$-like agonist sumatriptan has a significant effect in chronic tension-type headache. *Cephalalgia* 1992;12:375–9

13. Brennum J, Brinck T, Schriver L, *et al.* Sumatriptan has no clinically relevant effect in the treatment of episodic tension-type headache. *Eur J Neurol* 1996; 3:23–8

14. Olesen J. Responsiveness of non-IHS migraine and tension-type headache to sumatriptan. *Cephalalgia* 1997;17:559

# 8

# Secondary headaches

Laszlo L Mechtler and M Alan Stiles

## INTRODUCTION

The International Headache Society (IHS) classifies headaches (IHCD-II) into 14 major categories, subdivided into three broad groups: primary headache (categories 1–4), secondary headache (categories 5–12), and cranial neuralgias, central and primary facial pain and other headaches (categories 13–14) (Table 8.1). Secondary headaches represent a symptom of a pathological organic process and are associated with more than 316 disorders and illnesses. Secondary headaches can have serious and life-threatening causes, and up to 16% of annual emergency department (ED) visits are attributable to headache complaints. Fortunately, most headache complaints are due to primary headache disorders, such as migraine and tension-type headaches.

Headache is a common medical complaint, experienced by 75% of the American population, with over 5% seeking medical aid. The relative rarity of secondary headaches raises concern about the need for routine neuroimaging studies, especially when the neurologic examination is normal. Although practice guidelines have been developed, these guidelines were not designed to supersede clinical judgment when dealing with individual patients. The reality of patient and physician behavior in the present medical/legal milieu has resulted in the overuse of neuroimaging. Nevertheless, one cannot minimize a patient's anxiety in regard to a dramatic and disabling pain syndrome. This fear is amplified when children have severe headaches. Furthermore, managed-care systems often dictate which, if any, studies can be performed on their members. Therefore, the cost-to-benefit ratio of performing a study is tempered by the medical and legal implications of omitting the study.

## 'RED FLAGS'

The most common reason patients seek help at the ED is because of either their 'first or worst headache,' a frightening accompaniment (fever, confusion, focal neurological deficit) or treatment

**Table 8.1** ICHD-II headache classification. Reproduced from reference 1 with permission from Blackwell Publishing

| | |
|---|---|
| *Part one: The primary headaches* | |
| 1 | Migraine |
| 2 | Tension-type headache |
| 3 | Cluster headache and other trigeminal autonomic cephalalgias |
| 4 | Other primary headaches |
| *Part two: The secondary headaches* | |
| | Introduction |
| 5 | Headache attributed to head and/or neck trauma |
| 6 | Headache attributed to cranial or cervical vascular disorder |
| 7 | Headache attributed to non-vascular intracranial disorder |
| 8 | Headache attributed to a substance or its withdrawal |
| 9 | Headache attributed to infection |
| 10 | Headache attributed to disorder of homoeostasis |
| 11 | Headache or facial pain attributed to disorder of cranium, neck, eyes, ears, nose, sinuses, teeth, mouth or other facial or cranial structures |
| 12 | Headache attributed to psychiatric disorder |
| *Part three: Cranial neuralgias, central and primary facial pain and other headaches* | |
| 13 | Cranial neuralgias and central causes of facial pain |
| 14 | Other headache, cranial neuralgia, central or primary facial pain |

failure for a severe chronic headache (last-straw syndrome)[1,2]. Diagnostic alarms, or 'red flags,' help clinicians to lower the threshold in ordering neuroimaging studies. 'Red flags' include:

1. First or worst headache (thunderclap headache)
2. New-onset headache after age 50
3. Increasing headache frequency and severity
4. Chronic daily headaches unresponsive to treatment
5. Headaches always on the same side
6. Headaches following head trauma
7. Headaches with systemic illness (fever, stiff neck, rash)
8. Headaches associated with seizures
9. Headaches associated with atypical aura
10. Headaches associated with abnormal neurologic examination
11. New onset of headache in a human immunodeficiency virus (HIV) or cancer patient
12. Headaches in patients with neurocutaneous syndromes
13. Headaches precipitated by exertion, strain or positional changes

## PEDIATRIC 'RED FLAGS'

Of adults with headache who present to EDs, 16–20% have secondary headaches, as compared with 77% of all children who present to the ED. Of these children 45% suffer from secondary headaches due to neurologic causes[3]. 'Red flags' in children differ from the usual warning signs in adults and include:

1. Persistent headaches of less than 6 months' duration that do not respond to medical treatment;
2. Headaches associated with an abnormal neurologic finding, especially if accompanied by papilledema, nystagmus or gait or motor abnormalities;
3. Persistent headaches associated with a negative family history of migraine;
4. Persistent headaches associated with substantial episodes of confusion, disorientation or emesis;
5. Headaches that repeatedly awaken a child from sleep or occur immediately on awakening;
6. Family and medical history of disorders that predispose to CNS lesions and clinical laboratory findings that suggest CNS involvement.

## NEUROIMAGING

The United States Headache Consortium Report was unable to make any evidence-based recommendations with regard to the relative sensitivity of magnetic resonance (MR) imaging compared computerized tomography (CT) in evaluating migraine or other non-acute headache[5]. In the past, the advantage of CT was its cost, but over the last several years there has been a gradual decrease in reimbursement rate for MR imaging. CT is more sensitive than MR imaging in acute trauma, acute subarachnoid hemorrhage (within 24 h) and when MR imaging is contraindicated. MR imaging is more sensitive than CT in detecting neoplastic disease, cervical medullary lesions, pituitary disorders, and vascular diseases, including subdural hematomas, AVMs, ischemic disease, venous infarctions, dissections, aneurysms, and subarachnoid hemorrhages (after 72 h). Intracranial hypo- and hypertension are also better evaluated by MR imaging with and without gadolinium. Resolution and sensitivity in MR imaging has improved via larger magnet size, paramagnetic contrast and the selection of acquisition sequences for specific pathologic indications. Newer vascular imaging packages, such as MR angiography and MR venography, have also improved the sensitivity of MR imaging. CT angiography has recently been able to detect aneurysms greater than 2 mm and may be used as a screening tool instead of MR angiography.

In 1994, the American Academy of Neurology (AAN) provided a guideline for the use of neuroimaging in patients with headache and a normal neurologic examination (Quality Standard Subcommittee of the American Academy of Neurology, 1994)[6]. The consensus of the AAN (1994) was that 'the routine imaging in adult patients with recurrent headaches that have been defined as migraines – including those with visual auras (with no recent change in pattern, no history of seizures and no neurological signs or symptom)… is not warranted.' In patients with atypical headache patterns, history of seizures, and abnormal examinations, there is insufficient evidence to define the role of neuroimaging. As headaches account for approximately 4% of all outpatient visits, the final decision is left to the physician on a case-by-case basis. MR imaging is more sensitive in secondary headache of pregnancy, which may be caused by cardiovascular disease, sinus thombosis, pituitary apoplexia, DIC, or emboli, keeping in mind that contrast should be avoided.

## DIAGNOSTIC TESTING

When headaches fit the IHS criteria for migraine, diagnostic testing is usually unnecessary. However, when the headache is suspected to be due to an underlying pathology, diagnostic assays are of utmost importance. Erythrocyte sedimentation rate and C-reactive protein assay are the most commonly ordered diagnostic tests in the evaluation of secondary headaches when temporal arteritis is suspected. Auto-immune disorders, such as lupus or rheumatoid arthritis, can be ruled out with erythrocyte sedimentation rate, rheumatoid factor, and antineucleotide antibody assays. Mononucleosis testing should be done with a Monospot if the patient is a teenager. Electroencephalogram is not a useful diagnostic test unless headaches are associated with a loss of consciousness, confusion, or atypical aura reminiscent of epileptic conditions. Imaging followed by lumbar puncture can be advantageous if the patient has documented or suspected meningitis, encephalitis, leptomeningeal disease, subarachnoid hemorrhage, or cerebrospinal fluid pressure fluctuations. Finally, toxicology screens, arterial blood gases, complete blood count with differential, prolactin level, thyroid stimulating hormone level, liver functions tests, human immunodeficiency tests and carbon monoxide exposure tests can all be useful in determining the primary cause for the headache.

## DIFFERENTIAL DIAGNOSIS

The differential diagnosis of secondary headaches is quite extensive, but from a clinical perspective, the temporal course or pattern of headache presentation

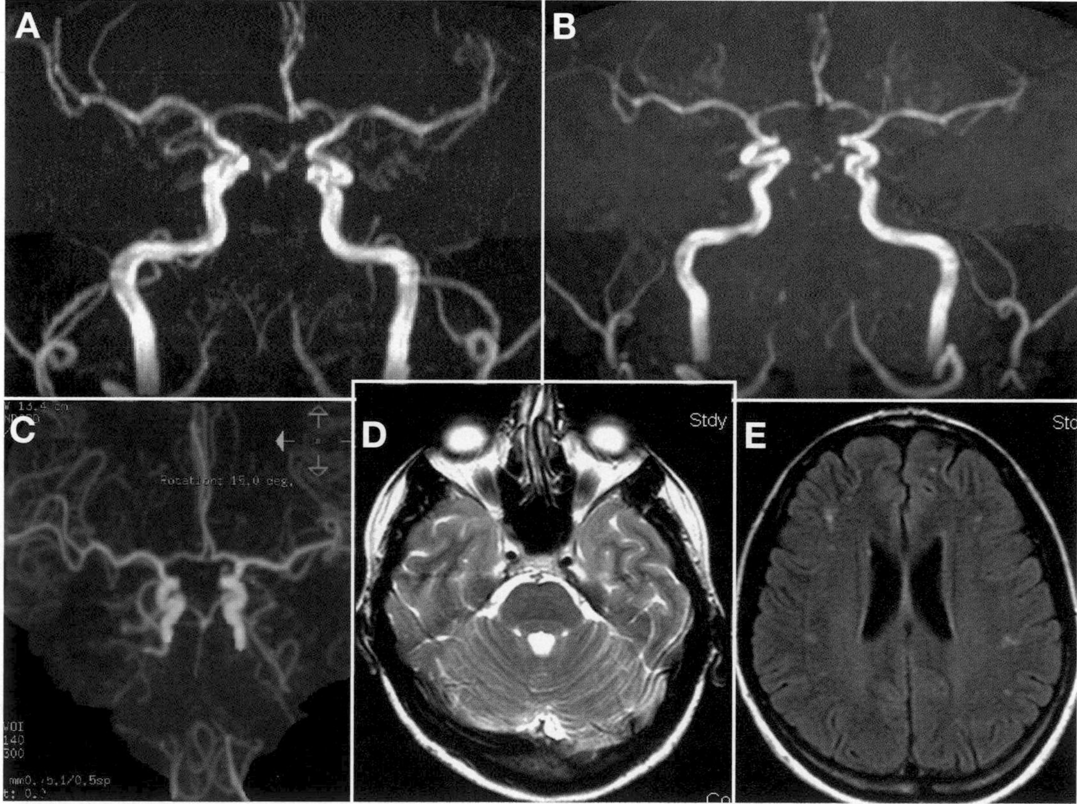


**Figure 8.1** A 34-year-old woman with a severe biocciptital throbbing headache associated with nausea, vertigo, and diplopia. Patient has a history of lupus. A and B. MR angiography shows an absent basilar artery. C. CT angiography confirms basilar occlusion. D. T2-weighted axial MR images through the brainstem shows no evidence of ischemic infarction within the brainstem, although the normal signal void within the basilar artery is absent. E. FLAIR axial MR images show corticomedullary white matter changes probably reflecting areas of ischemic demyelinization or gliosis

is essential for diagnosis and treatment. Three categories most frequently used include:

1. 'First or worst' abrupt-onset headache
2. Subacute-onset headache
3. Insidious-onset headache

I. The differential diagnosis of the acute or *severe new-onset headache* (the 'first or worst' headache) include:
   a. Migraine ('crash,' thunderclap variant)
   b. Cluster
   c. Hemorrhage
      i. Subarachnoid hemorrhage
      ii. Parenchymal hemorrhage
      iii. Epidural/subdural hematoma
      iv. Pituitary apoplexia
      v. Hemorrhage in tumor
         1. Melanoma
         2. Oligodendroglioma
      vi. Internal carotid/vertebrobasilar dissection
      vii. Ischemic cerebrovascular disease
      viii. Cerebral venous thrombosis
      ix. Acute hypertension
         1. Pheochromocytoma
         2. Pre-eclampsia
      x. Acute obstructive hydrocephalus
         1. Herniation syndrome
            a. Tonsillar
            b. Subfalcine
            c. Uncal
      xi. Non-neural
         1. Acute glaucoma
         2. Sinusitis (sphenoid, frontal)
         3. Head trauma

II. A subacute pattern of pain buildup occurs over hours and/or days and may be associated with intermittent periods of complete or relatively complete freedom from pain. Conditions associated with *subacute-onset headaches* include:
   a. Intracranial hypertension
   b. Arteriovenous malformations
   c. Withdrawal headaches (analgesic, ergotamine, triptan)
   d. Subdural hematoma (post-traumatic or spontaneous)
   e. Intracranial hypotension (spontaneous, post-traumatic)
   f. Cerebral vasculitis
   g. Brain tumor (primary, metastatic)
   h. Brain abscess/CNS infection
   i. Cervical spine disease
   j. Dental, temporomandibular disorder calvarial disease
   k. Sinusitis
   l. Whiplash injury

III. *Insidious-onset headaches* frequently evolve into chronic daily headaches, although they tend to be slowly progressive in nature when due to organic causes. Investigation is essential if there is a history of progressive pain. If there is no apparent progression, neuro-diagnostic testing may only be prudent when symptoms are disabling and/or the pain does not respond to treatment. Conditions associated with insidious onset headaches include:
   a. Intracranial hypotension or hypertension
   b. Fungal, parasiticor neoplastic, sarcoid-related meningoencephalitis
   c. Sinusitis (i.e. sphenoid, frontal)
   d. Vasculitis (i.e. temporal arteritis)
   e. Cerebral vein thrombosis
   f. Metabolic disorders
      i. Drug induced ($H_2$ blocker, nitrates, NSAID)
      ii. Hypercarbia-hypoxia
      iii. Hyperthyroidism
      iv. Carbon monoxide poisoning
   g. Brain neoplasm (slow-growing)
   h. Postconcussion syndrome (post-traumatic)

## HEADACHES IN THE ELDERLY

Secondary headaches in patients over the age of 50 present a challenge to the clinician. Only 2% of migraineurs have their first headache over the age of 50. In addition, as the incidence of primary headaches declines with age, secondary headaches increase with advancing age. Although neoplasms may cause headaches in all age groups, they are far more prevalent in patients over the age of 50. The common causes of headaches beginning late in life include primary and secondary neoplasms, temporal arteritis, drug-induced headaches, trigeminal neuralgia, cervicogenic headache, Parkinson's disease, cerebrovascular disease, postherpetic neuralgia and headaches associated with systemic diseases.

## HEENT HEADACHE

Category 2 in the IHS classification describes headache-associated disorders of the cranium, neck, eyes, ears, nose, sinuses, teeth or other facial and cranial structures. This group includes two disorders that are often mistakenly believed to be associated with headaches: (a) temporomandibular disorders (TMD) and (b) chronic sinusitus. Seventy percent of the population may have TMD, but it is estimated that less than 5% of patients have associated headaches. The most common cause of pain related to TMD is a myofascial syndrome. Sinus disease is a disorder that is erroneously implicated as a cause of headaches. Headache and facial pain usually occur with the acute stage of purulent sinusitis supported by diagnostic studies (X-ray, CT/MRI). Chronic sinusitis is not validated as a cause of headaches or facial pain unless it relapses into the acute stage. In addition, up to 88% percent of patients presenting with recurrent 'sinus headaches' meet IHS criteria for migraines or migrainous headaches.

## CRANIAL NEURALGIAS

Cranial neuralgias are listed in IHS Category 13. Neuralgia is defined as an intense, burning or stabbing pain caused by irritation or damage to a nerve. Two general forms of neuralgia are known, one idiopathic

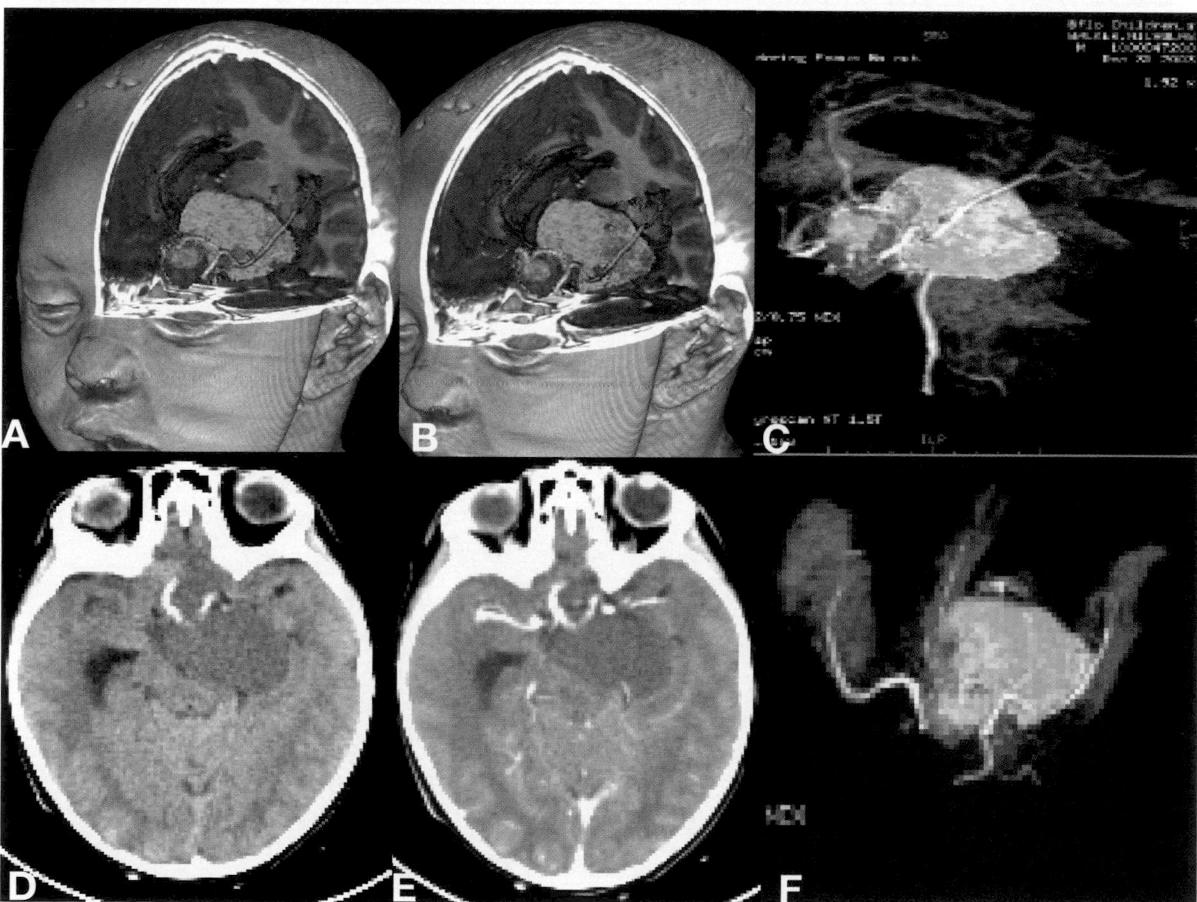


**Figure 8.2** A 4-year-old with progressive headaches, papilledema and and obstructive hydrocephalus. (A), (B) and (C) show a 3-D reconstruction of a craniopharyngioma: green represents tumor, blue represents calcification and red is the surrounding vasculature. (D) and (E) demonstrate a non-contrast and contrast CT of a suprasellar hypodensity as well as a right temporal horn enlargement. (F) is an anterior posterior view of the tumor in close proximity to the circle of Willis. Reproduced with kind permission of Ron Alberico

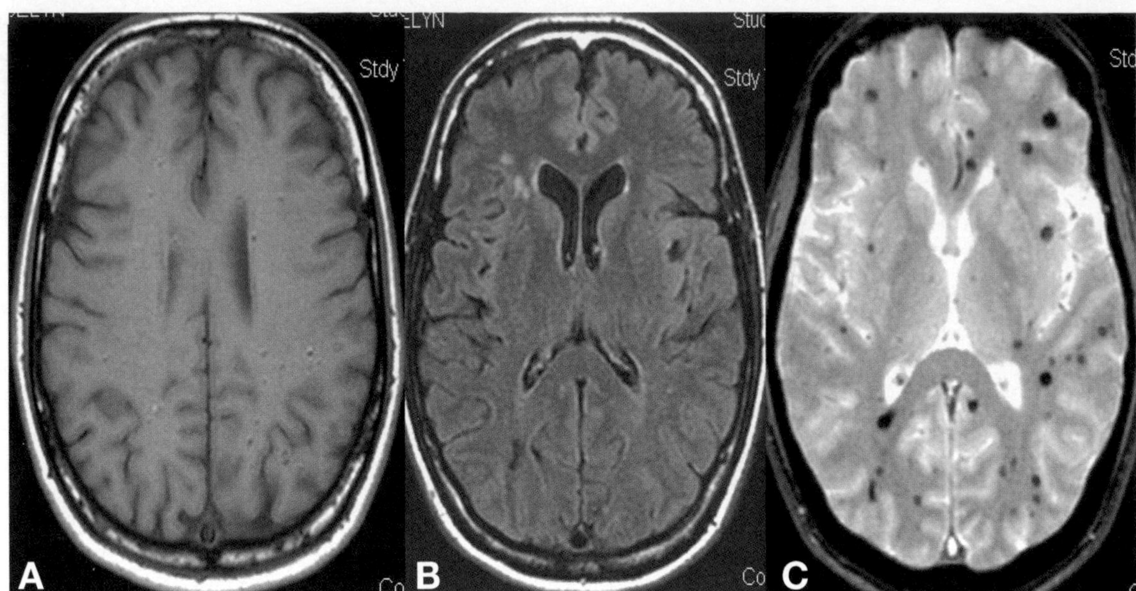


**Figure 8.3** A 38-year-old female with a family history of vascular malformations presents with episodic diffuse headaches, photophobia and nausea. Neurologic examination was normal. Although symptoms were highly suggestive of migraine, patient underwent a MRI because of the family history. A. T1-weighted non-contrast axial image shows multiple punctate hypointensities with a partial rim of hyperintensity. B. FLAIR axial images are relatively unrevealing except for some non-specific ischemic changes. C. The study of choice is a gradient echo MR image showing multiple hemosiderin-laden small bleeds consistent with the diagnosis of hereditary cavernous hemangioma

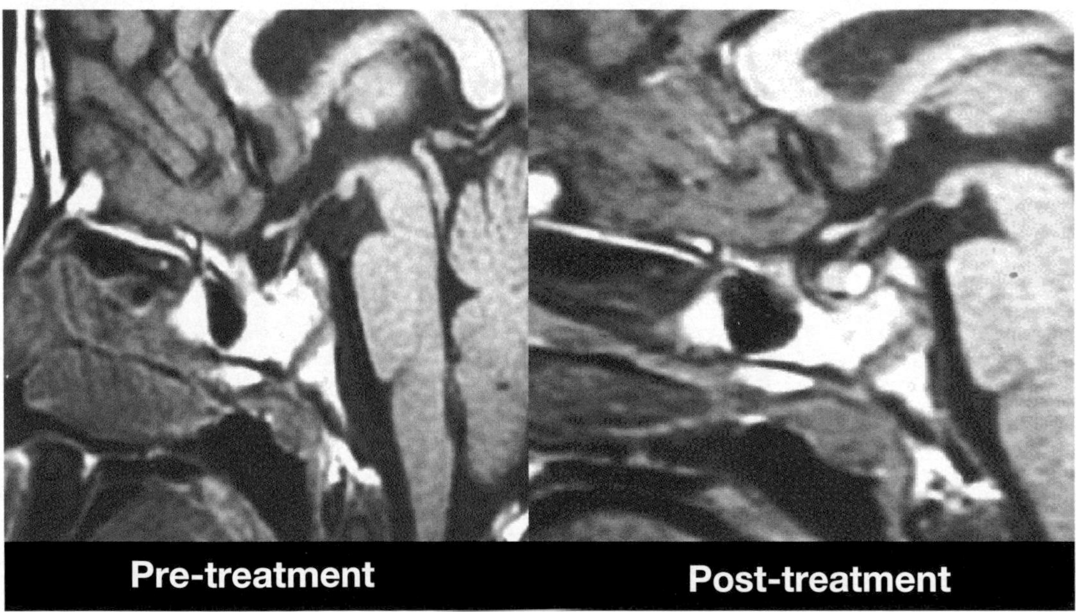


**Figure 8.4** A 9-year-old male patient with idiopathic intracranial hypertension (pseudotumor cerebri) initially presented with loss of appetite and frontal headache that over 4 months progressed to daily headaches with visual obscurations. Neurologic examination was normal as was the fundoscopic exam. Pre-treatment T1-weighted sagittal MR image shows a partially empty sella. Post-treatment T1-weighted sagittal MR image, obtained 4 months after three lumbar punctures, shows a re-expanded pituitary gland within the sella turcica associated with improvement of clinical symptoms. Reproduced with permission from Suzuki H, Takanashi J, Kobayashi K, *et al*. MR imaging of idiopathic intracranial hypertension. *Am J Neuroradiol* 2001;22:196–9

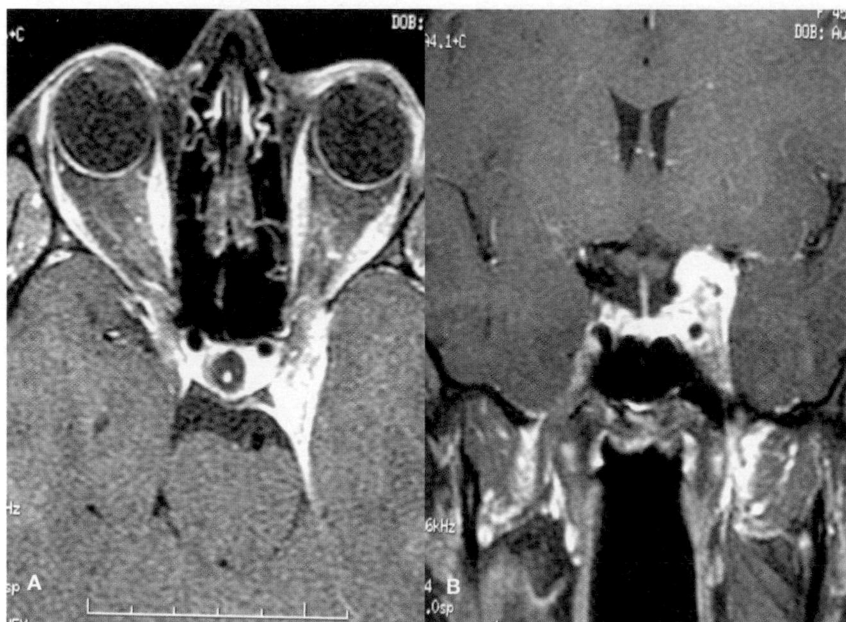

**Figure 8.5** Meningioma infiltrating the left cavernous sinus causing a left parasellar syndrome with supraorbital pain and partial third nerve palsy. A. T1-weighted fat suppression (STIR) MR image in the axial plane with gadolinium (Gd) contrast. B. Coronal T1-weighted Gd contrast MR image with extension of the tumor into the suprasellar cistern

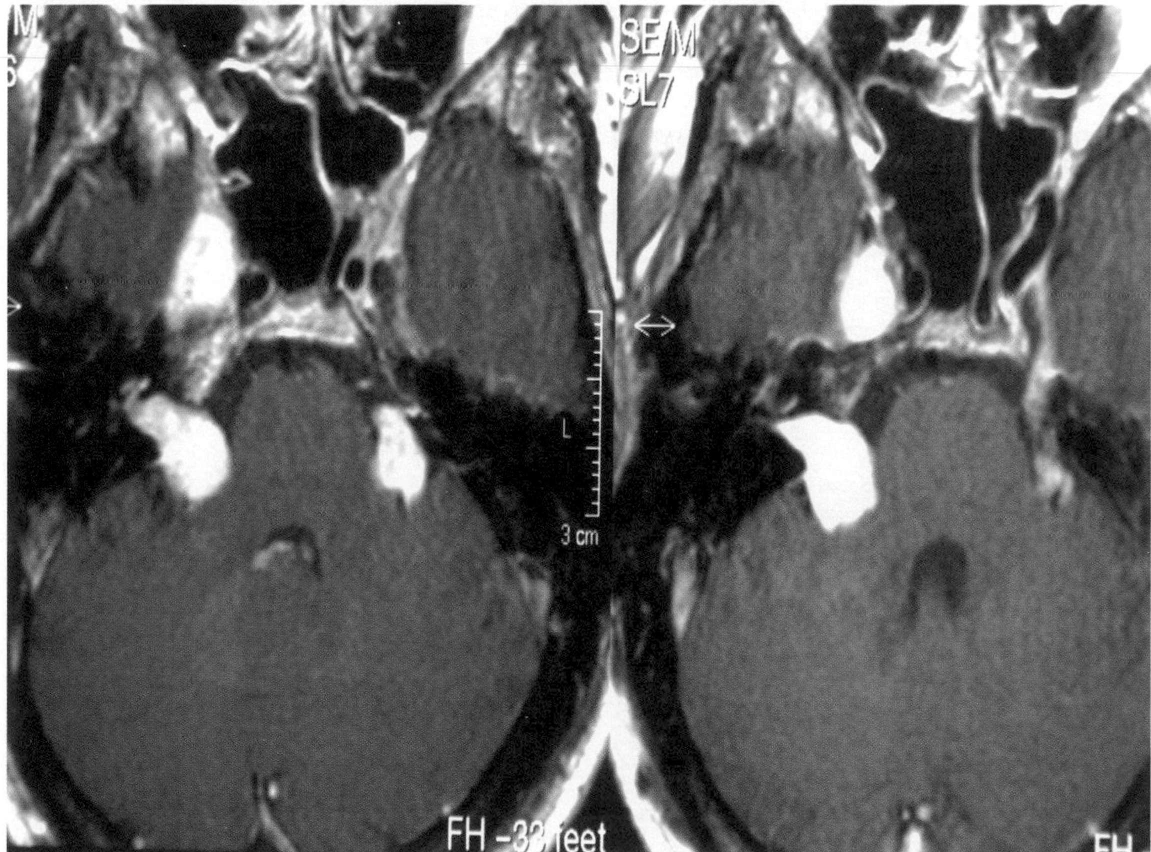

**Figure 8.6** Multiple schwannomas in a patient with neurofibromatosis-2. Bilateral vestibular and right Meckel's cave schwannomas are evident on these T1-weighted axial contrast MR images. Patient presented with trigeminal paresthesias and neuralgic pain, as well as hearing loss

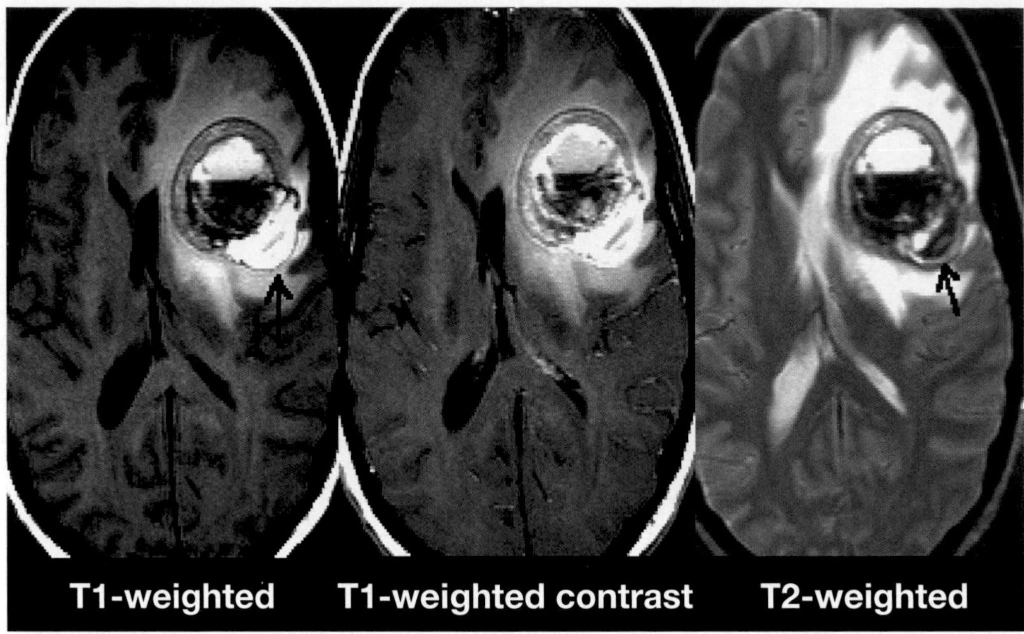


**Figure 8.7** Axial MRI study shows an encapsulated single hemorrhagic metastasis within the left frontal lobe that is associated with vasogenic edema, ventricular and sulcal effacement, as well as early midline shift. Patient is a 36-year-old female who presented with severe throbbing left frontal headache with nausea that was acute in onset. Past medical history is significant for cutaneous melanoma resected 5 years ago. Patient's headaches resolved after complete resection and external beam radiation

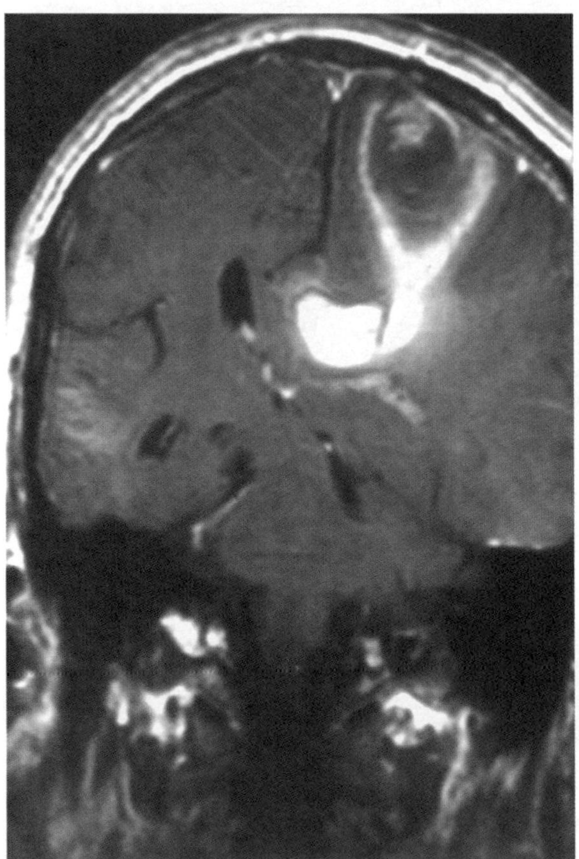

**Figure 8.8** 49-year-old woman with a past medical history of melanoma presented with a severe throbbing but continuous headache over the vertex for 48 h. Coronal T1-weighted contrast MRI shows a hemorrhagic metastasis with subfalcine (cingulate) herniation with midline shift. Postoperatively the headache resolved

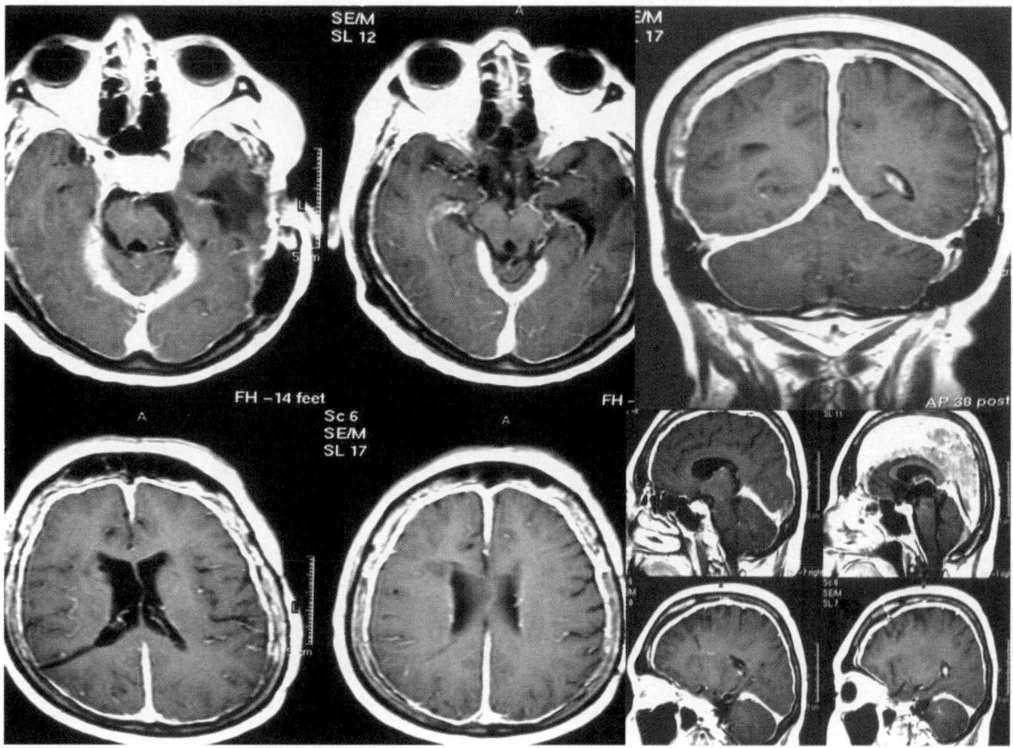


**Figure 8.9** Gadolinium contrast MR images in the axial, coronal and sagittal plane demonstrating diffuse pachymeningeal thickening and enhancement. Patient is a 40-year-old male complaining of postural headaches after resection of left middle fossa meningioma. In patients with positional or exertional headaches, contrast studies may be diagnostic in intracranial hypotension

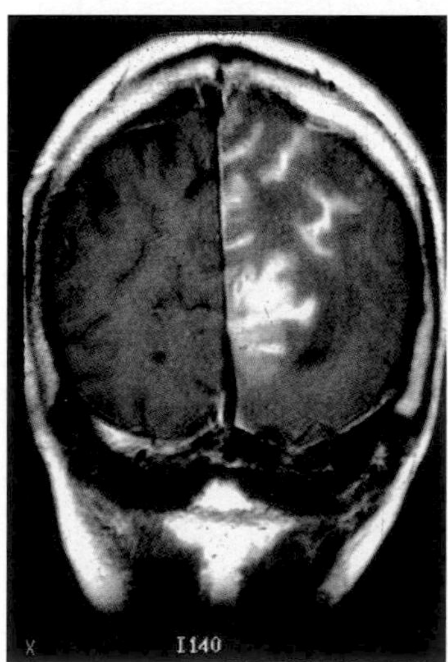


**Figure 8.10** A 65-year-old with a 2-year history of bronchogenic carcinoma presented with continuous progressive occipital headache that was unresponsive to medication. Coronal T1-weighted contrast MRI studies confirmed enhancement within the sulci consistent with leptomeningeal disease or carcinomatosis. Lumbar puncture confirmed diagnosis. Headache responded to steroids and external beam radiation

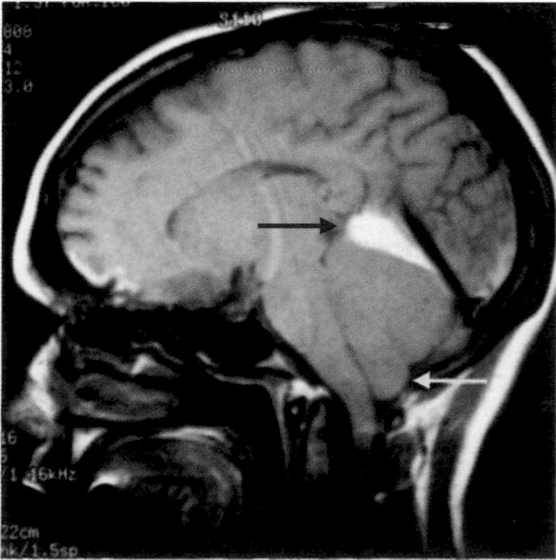

**Figure 8.11** A 34-year-old male status post closed head injury 2 weeks ago complained of a dull occipital headache that worsened with head flexion. Sagittal non-contrast MR image showed an acute subdural hematoma (red arrow) below the tentorium cerebelli causing early tonsillar herniation and increased posterior fossa pressure (yellow arrow)

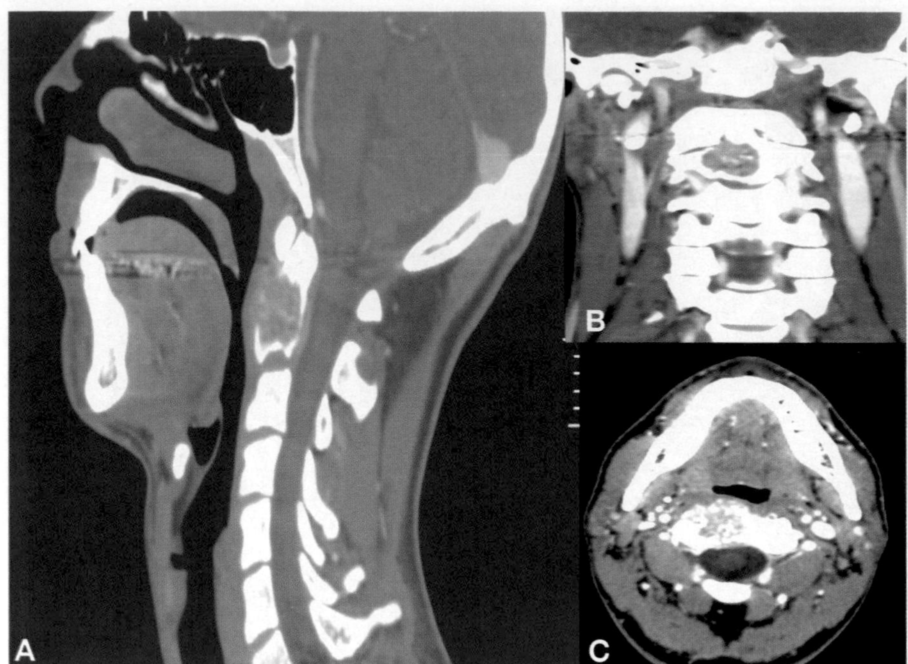


**Figure 8.12** CT images show in multiple planes (A sagittal, B coronal and C axial) a destructive C2 vertebral body metastasis in 50-year-old with a history of broncho-alveolar carcinoma who presented with occipital neuralgia on the left as well as rotational neck pain. Patient responded to external beam radiation

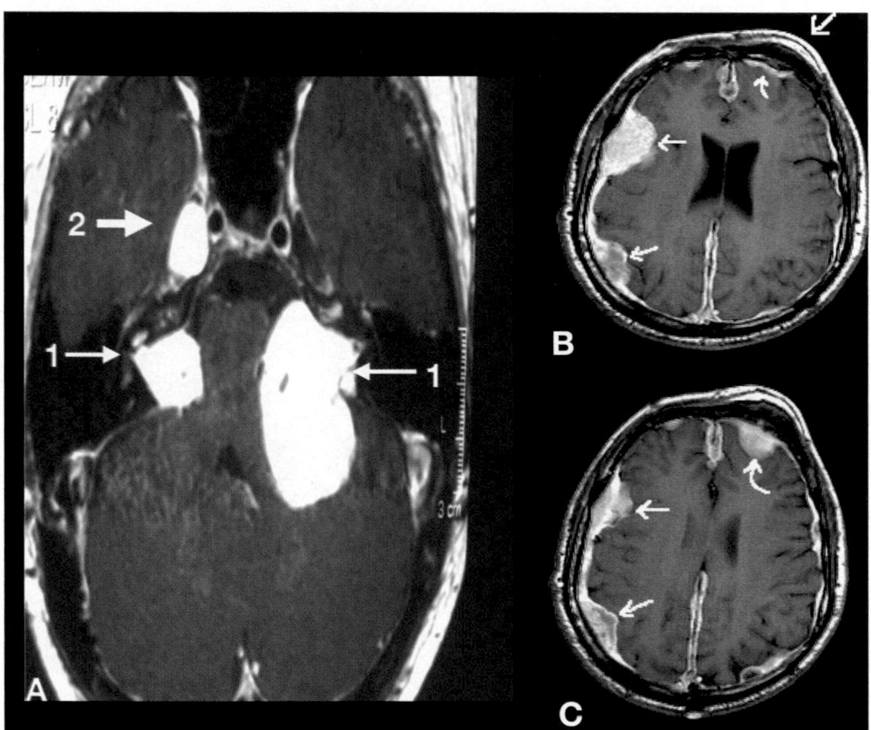


**Figure 8.13** A 41-year-old patient with chronic headaches, hearing loss and right facial numbness had evidence on MRI of neurofibromatosis type 2. Also known as "MISME" (multiple inherited schwannomas, meningiomas and ependymomas) this is an autosomal dominant disorder involving deletions on chromosome 22. Axial contrast T1-weighted MRI shows bilateral enhancing vestibular schwannomas (1) and a right trigeminal schwannoma (2). B and C show multiple en plaque, falx and convexity meningiomas. The left frontal convexity meningioma is extending through the calvarium causing localized pain (intraosseus meningioma)

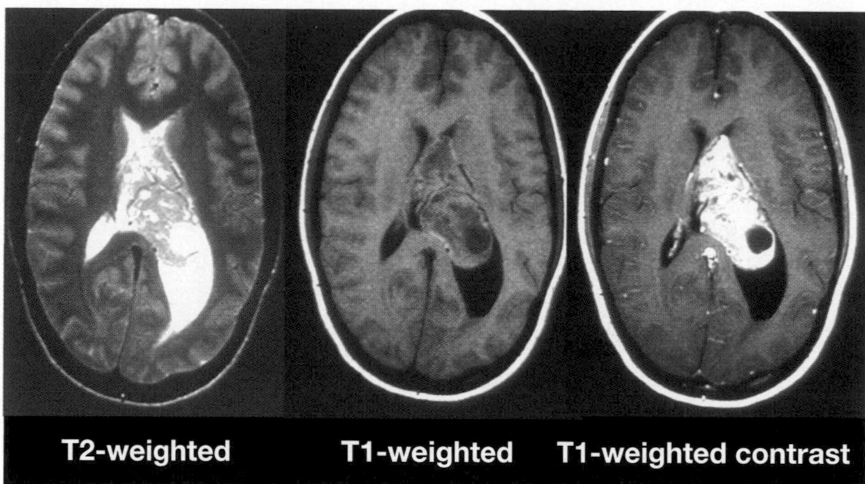


**Figure 8.14** Heterogeneous enhancing intraventricular mass with a focal obstructive hydrocephalus of the left occipital horn in a 45-year-old female. Presenting symptom was a throbbing, intractable headache with nausea, initially intermittent, then chronic. Initial diagnosis was migraine; postoperatively, a tumor was consistent with neurocytoma

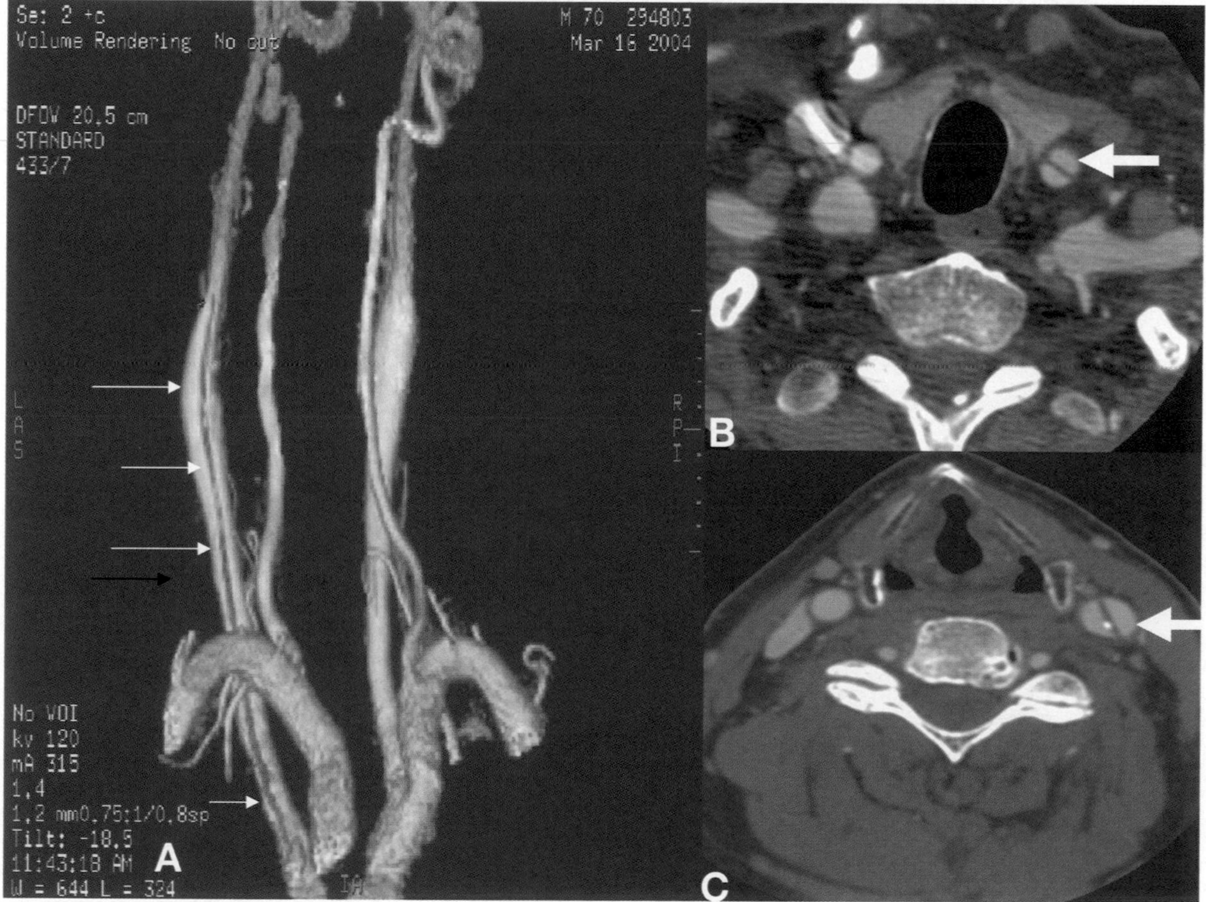


**Figure 8.15** A 70-year-old male with a 1-week history of left temporal and cervical pain associated with a Horner's pupil. No history of trauma. CT angiogram with volume rendering (A) shows a full length carotid dissection. Axial CT ( B and C) shows a false lumen. Patient also complained of upper back pain and was found to have a dissecting aorta, which was repaired. Reproduced with kind permission of Ron Alberico

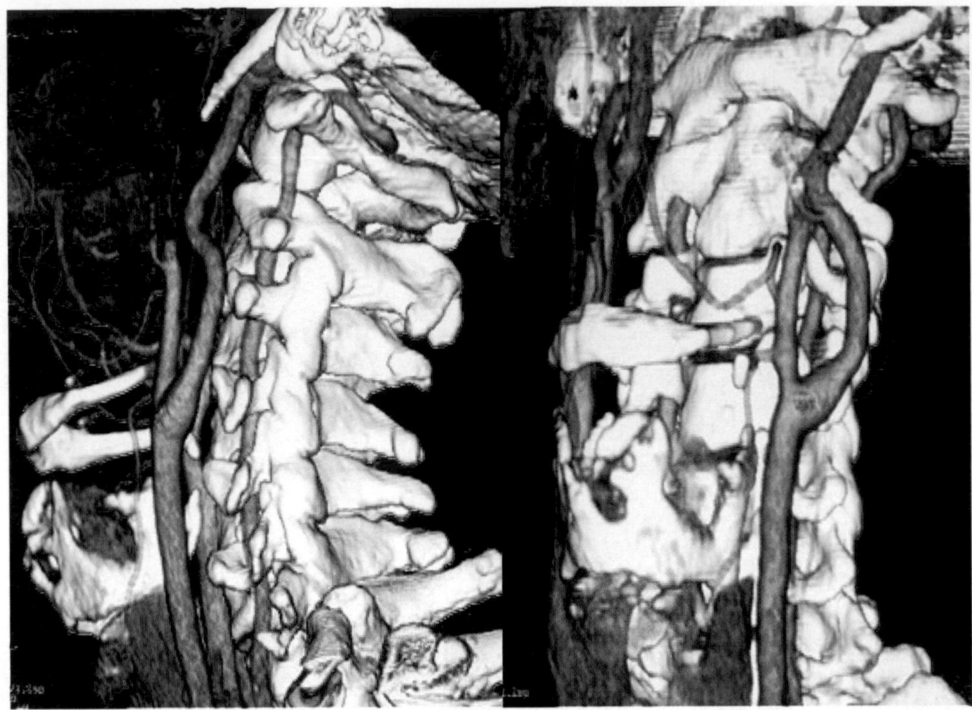

**Figure 8.16** An advantage of volume-rendered CT angiogram is that it shows excellent vascular soft tissue and bony detail. Reproduced with kind permission of Ron Alberico

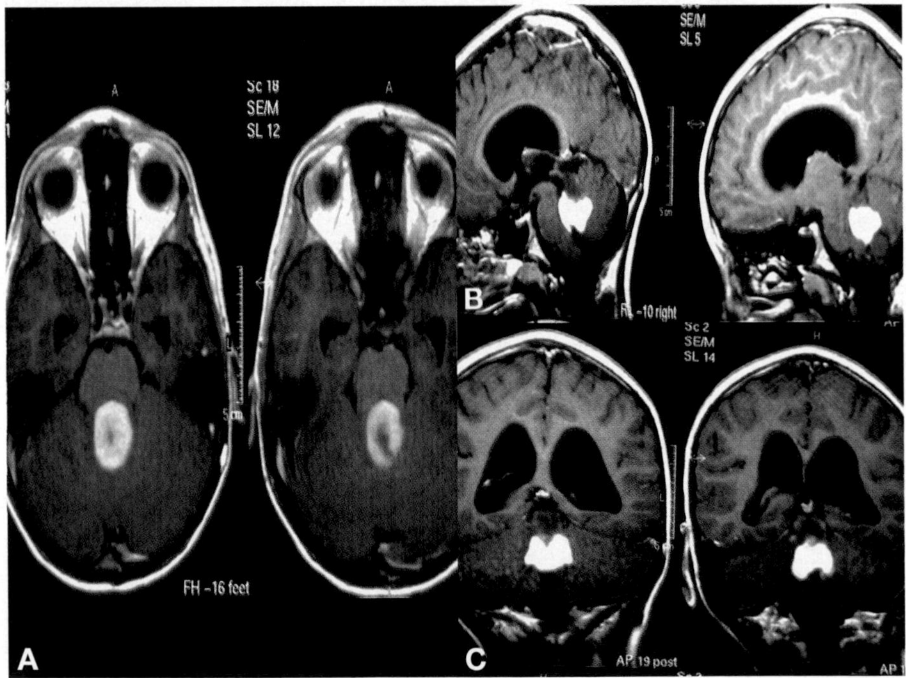


**Figure 8.17** An 18-year-old male with contrast-enhancing mass within the fourth ventricle causing obstructive hydrocephalus. Symptoms included a subacute diffuse headache with nausea and vomiting. T1-weighted axial (A), sagittal (B) and coronal (C) post-gadolinium studies show an intraventricular mass obstructing the fourth ventricle. On examination, the patient had papilledema, which is far more commonly seen with posterior fossa masses

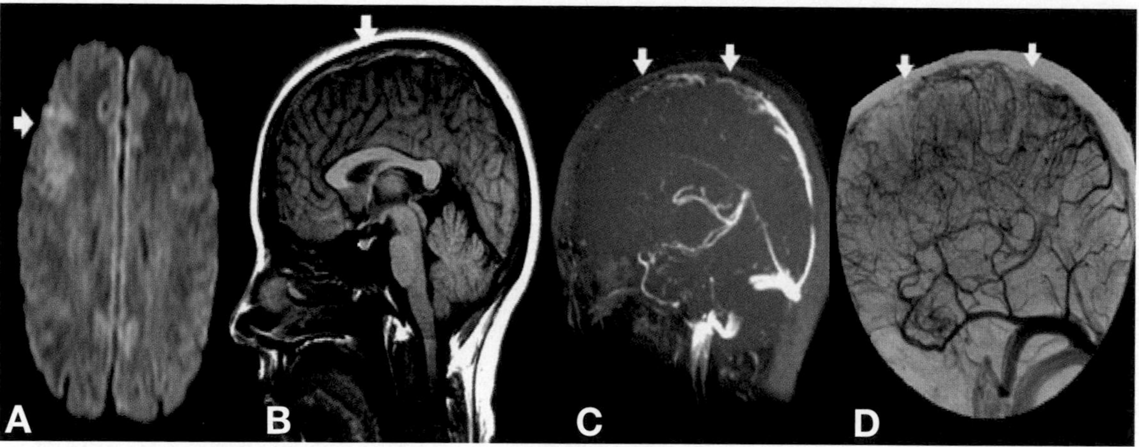


**Figure 8.18** A 32-year-old woman who presented with a severe headache and seizure. Diffusion weighted images (A) confirm a acute right frontal lobe infarct not in the typical arterial distribution. T1 and T2 weighted images were normal within the first 24 h of presentation. T1-weighted sagittal (B) images showed an increased signal representing a thrombus within the superior sagittal sinus. MR venogram (C) and venous phase angiogram (D) support the diagnosis of superior sagittal thrombosis. Risk factors for venous thrombosis include: dehydration, pregnancy, oral contraceptives, trauma, DIC, neoplasms, hypercoagable states, infections and idiopathic. Reproduced with kind permission of Rohit Bakshi

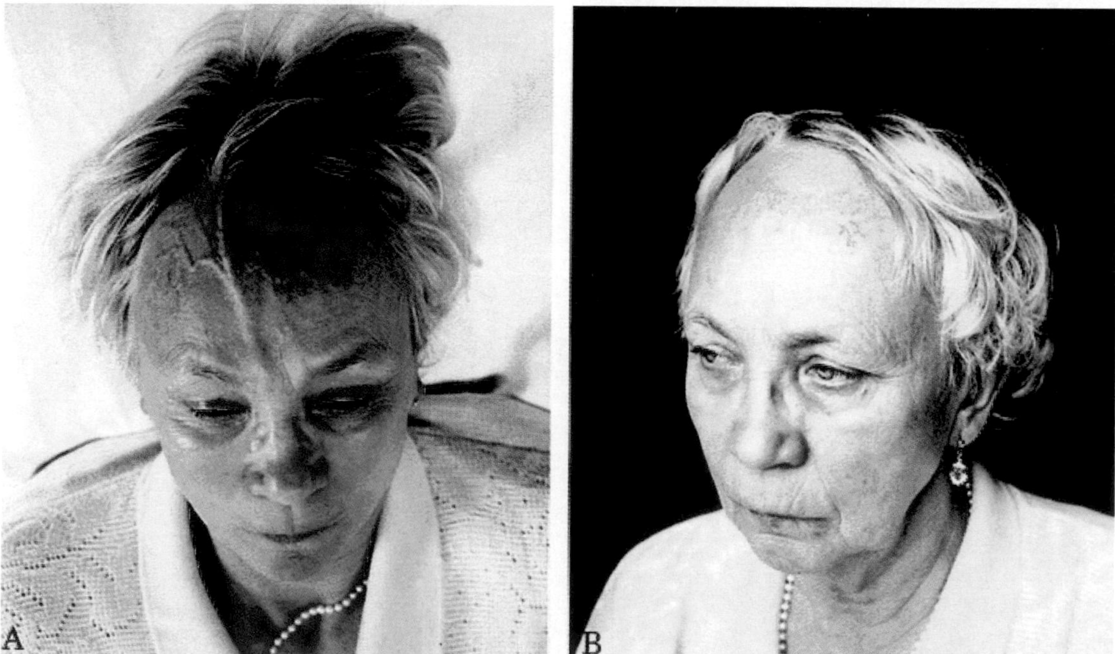


**Figure 8.19** A 62-year-old woman with a 2-month history of headache, impaired vision and phosphenes. Patient was found to have a thrombosis of the posterior superior sagittal sinus and both transverse sinuses. Patient recanalized partially with anticoagulation. On initial examination patient's forehead veins were swollen, presenting as a 'caput medusae' when in a supine position (A), but not when she was sitting (B). This phenomenon may be explained by the hindered venous flow along the internal jugular vein, which is the predominant venous drainage in the supine position. In the upright position the spinal epidural veins may open as an additional drainage pathway. Reproduced with permission from Meyer BU, Hoffman KT. Caput medusae after sinus venous thrombosis. *Neurology* 2001;57:1376

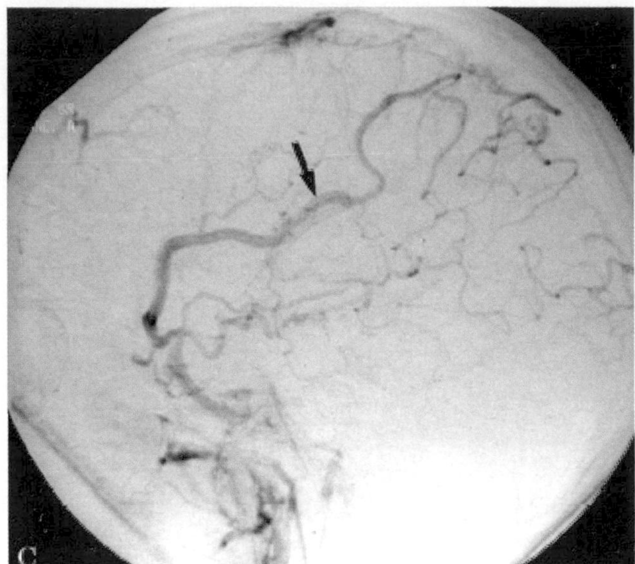

**Figure 8.20** Venous drainage in the angiogram (supine position, C) revealed drainage of the superior sagittal sinus along the superficial middle cerebral vein and along the emissary veins through the diploe. Reproduced with permission from Meyer BU, Hoffman KT. Caput medusae after sinus venous thrombosis. *Neurology* 2001;57:1376

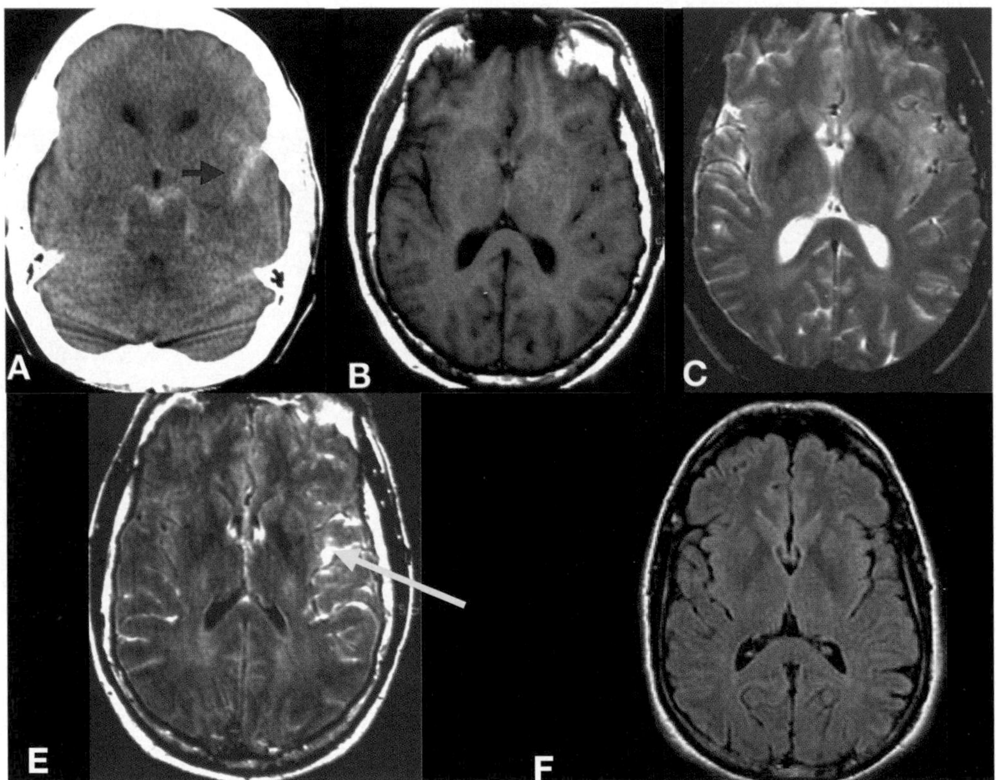


**Figure 8.21** A 30-year-male presenting with the 'worst headache of his life' was found to have subarachnoid hemorrhage (SAH) due to a left middle cerebral aneurysm rupture. CT (A) is the study of choice within 24 h of acute onset of symptoms when compared to MRI specifically T1(B) and T2(C)-weighted images. Red arrow points to hyperdensity within the Sylvian fissure representing blood. Fluid attenuated inversion recovery (FLAIR) sequence (E) is as sensitive as CT between 24–72 h and more sensitive after 72 h. Yellow arrow points to subarachnoid hyperintensity representing blood. A normal FLAIR (F) image is shown for comparison. FLAIR imaging is especially useful when SAH patients have symptoms 7 days prior to presenting to the emergency room or a physician. Reproduced with kind permission of Rohit Bakshi

and the other secondary. The prototype of cranial neuralgia is trigeminal neuralgia, which is characterized by a brief, electric-shock-like pain, frequently in the distribution of cranial nerves VII and VIII. Secondary causes of cranial neuralgias include tumors at the base of the skull, vascular compression, neuritis, multiple sclerosis, herpes zoster, sinus and dental disease and trauma. Glossopharyngeal and occipital neuralgia are well-defined cranial neuralgias.

## CONCLUSION

The final decision of whether to use diagnostic testing for patients with headaches lies in the clinical judgment of the treating physician. Patients presenting with the 'first or worst' headache and an abnormal neurologic examination should be investigated without hesitation. The patient's response to migraine-specific treatment should not be consid-

| Time | Probability % |
|---|---|
| Day 0 | 95 (Adams *et al.*, 1983) |
| Day 3 | 74 (Adams *et al.*, 1983) |
| 1 week | 50 (van Gijn and van Dongen, 1982) |
| 2 weeks | 30 (van Gijn and van Dongen, 1982) |
| 3 weeks | Almost 0 (van Gijn and van Dongen, 1982) |

Reproduced with permission from Evans RW. Headaches. In: Evans RW, ed. *Diagnostic Testing in Neurology*. Philadelphia: WB Saunders, 1999:9

**Figure 8.22** Approximate probability of recognizing an aneurysmal subarachnoid hemorrhage on CT scan after the initial event

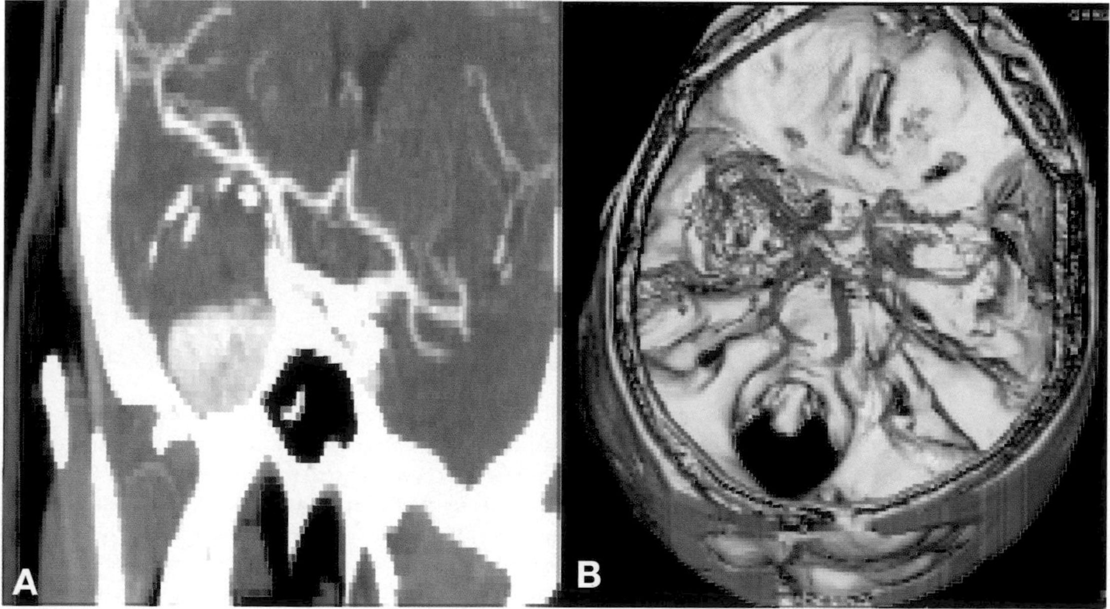


**Figure 8.23** Patient is a 60-year-old woman with intermittent migrainous type headache located to his right frontal/periorbital region. Recently headaches have increased in frequency and severity. Patient was found to have a giant left cavernous internal carotid artery aneurysm. CT angiogram (A) shows a left giant aneurysm, that is partially thrombosed and calcified. Patient underwent a coil occlusion with resolution of headaches. (B) Volume-rendered CT of the head with yellow representing an aneurysm

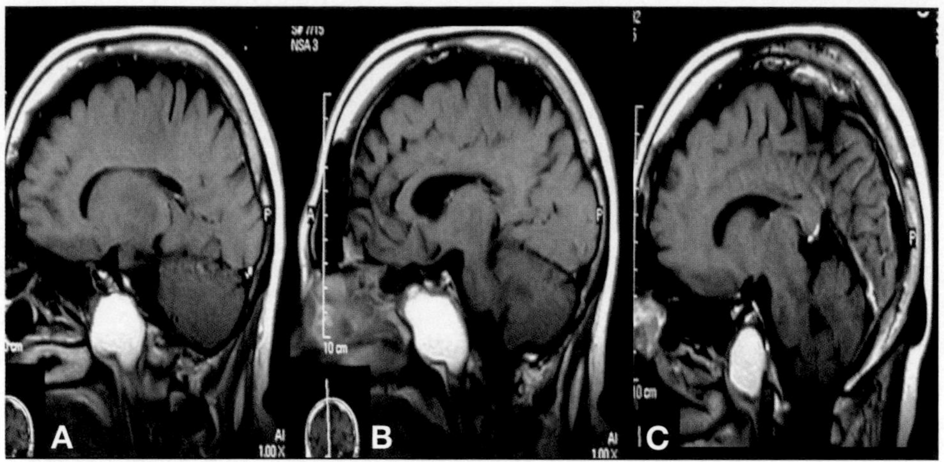


**Figure 8.24** Patient is a 40-year-old male complaining of a diffuse headache which is aggravated by bending and coughing. T1-weighted serial sagittal non-contrast MR images show a hyperintensity within the sphenoid sinus consistent with a mucocele. This is an expansile non-infectious lesion that causes symptoms by its mass effect

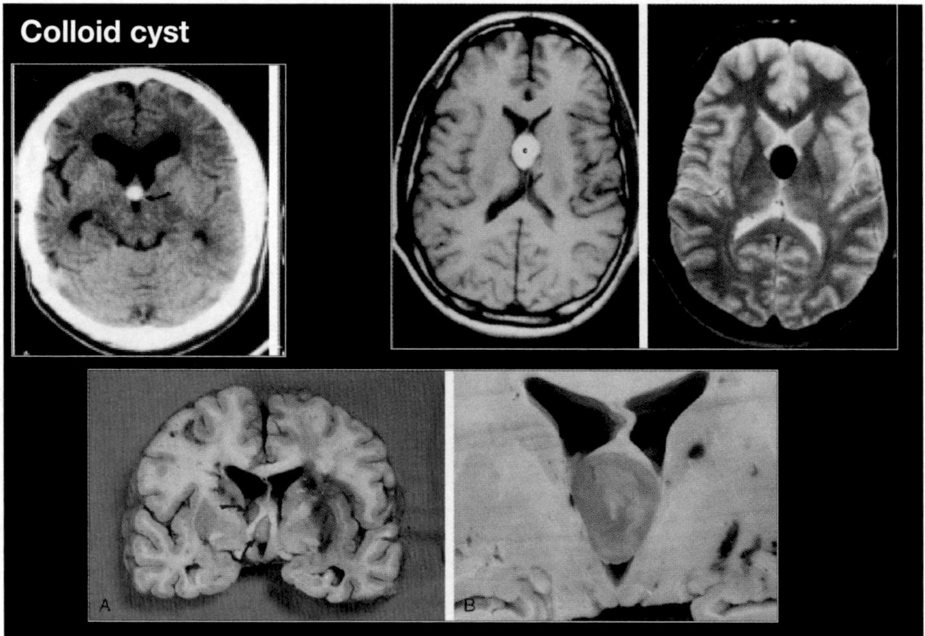


**Figure 8.25** The patient was a 36-year-old woman with a medical history significant for AIDS with multiple opportunistic infections, including *Pneumocystis carinii* and *Mycobacterium kanasii* pneumonias, cerebral toxoplasmosis, and cryptococcal meningitis as well as a history of a colloid cyst of the third ventricle detected by CT. She had recently been admitted to an outside hospital for unexplained fever and painful lower extremity edema. During treatment for acute-onset renal failure, the patient developed headache and nuchal rigidity. T1-weighted non-contast MRI shows a ovoid hyperintensity within the superior anterior third ventricle. T2-weighted images show just the opposite signal characteristics. Fixed brain. A, Coronal section shows elevation of the fornices and obstruction of the interventricular foramina of Monro by the colloid cyst (arrows). Bilateral multifocal acute hemorrhages are seen in the periventricular white matter. A hemorrhagic infarction in the left basal ganglia is seen. B, Cut surface of colloid cyst displays turbid, gelatinous material. The fornices are lifted and the third ventricle is expanded. Headache occurs in 68–100% of patients and is often the presenting symptom. Headaches are characterized as brief, lasting seconds to minutes, and are initiated, exacerbated, or relieved by a change in position. Reproduced with permission from Armao D, Castillo M, Chen H, Kwock L. Colloid cyst of the third ventricle: imaging-pathologic correlation. *Am J Neuroradiol* 2000;21:1470–7

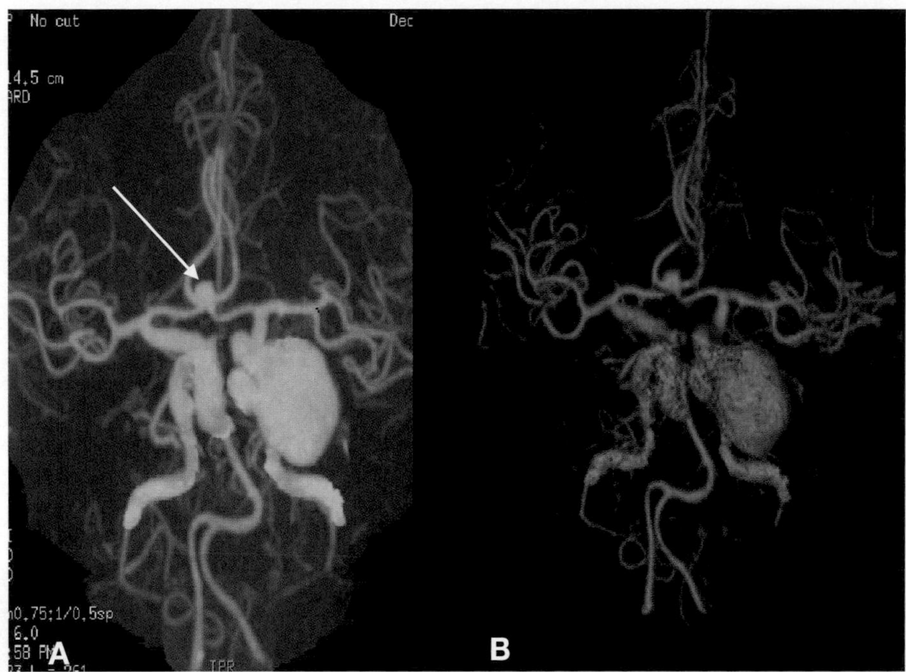


**Figure 8.26** A 32-year-old woman with a 6-month history of intermittent disabling left frontal-orbital headaches and a normal examination. (A) MR angiogram and 3-D volume-rendered MRA confirm a left internal carotid cavernous sinus giant aneurysm. In addition, aneurysms in the anterior communicating and in the right internal carotid arteries were found. 20% of aneurysms are multiple. Sentinel headaches occur in close to half of all patients with ruptured aneurysms. Sentinel headaches are migraine or headaches due to minor leaks

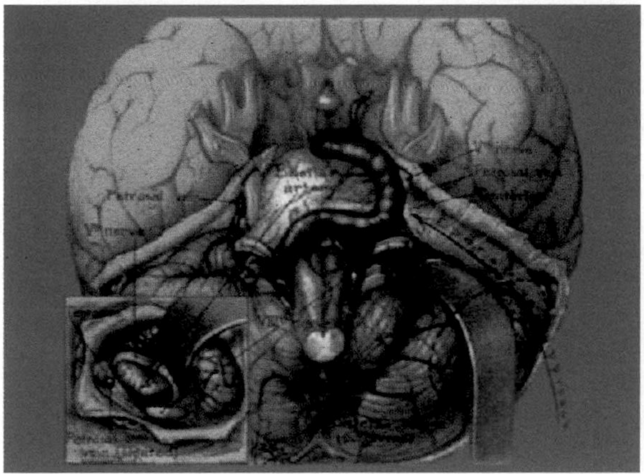

**Figure 8.27** Vascular compression theory for trigeminal neuralgia. One of the first surgical proponents of the vascular theory was Walter Dandy. In 1934, Dandy wrote, 'I believe no less responsible for the production of trigeminal neuralgia; these are the arteries and veins which impinge upon and frequently distort the sensory root. In the region of the sensory root the superior arterial branch forms a loop…as the artery hardens from advancing age, the nerve becomes indented by the arterial branch'. Reproduced from Dandy WE. Concerning the cause of trigeminal neuralgia. *Am J Surg* 1934;24:447–55, with permission from Excerpta Medica Inc

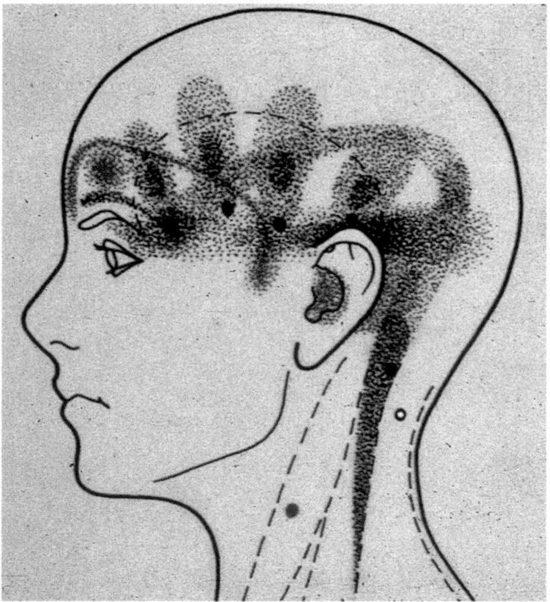

**Figure 8.28** Overlapping pain referral patterns from myofascial trigger points in various masticatory and cervical muscles produce typical unilateral or bilateral migraine or tension-type headache. Reproduced with kind permission of Bernadette Jaeger

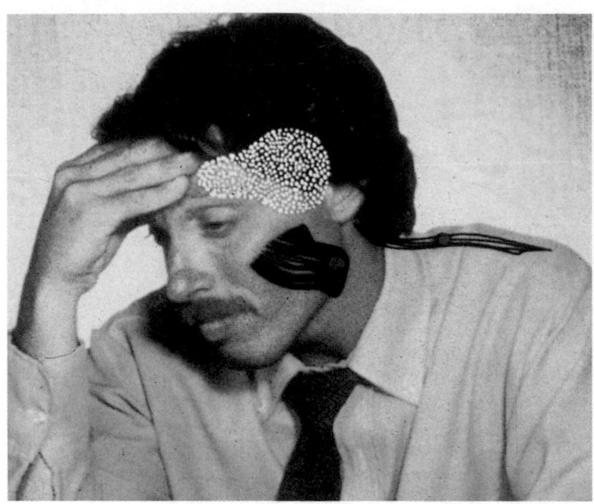

**Figure 8.29** Referred pain from superficial masseter and upper trapezius myofascial trigger points may produce unilateral or bilateral tension-type and migraine headache symptoms. Reproduced with kind permission of Bernadette Jaeger

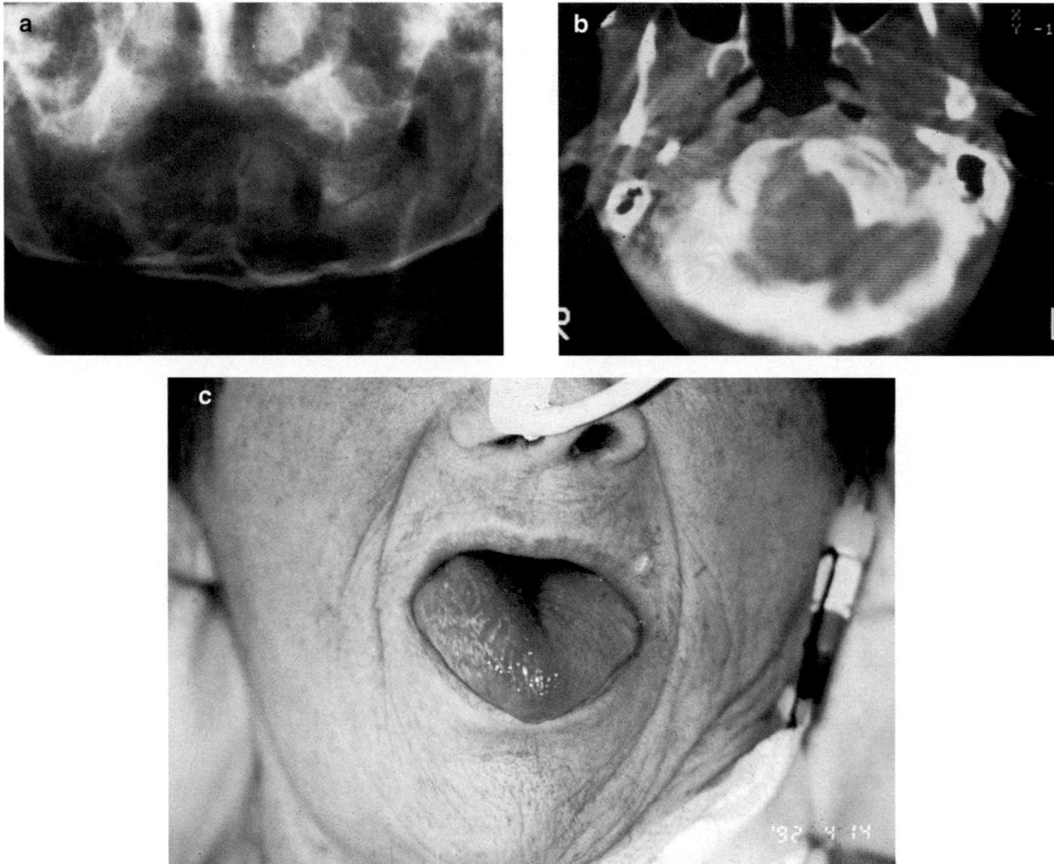


**Figure 8.30** (a), (b) and (c) belong to the same patient, a 67-year-old woman with severe, continuous left occipital pain and swallowing difficulties during the previous two weeks. The pain became unbearable with right suboccipital palpation or on neck rotation to the left. Neurologic examination showed a right twelfth nerve paralysis. She died suddenly several days after admission. Clinical diagnosis was 'right occipital condyle syndrome' secondary to a metastasis of unknown origin. (a) Posteroanterior skull radiograph with an inclination of 30° showing an osteolytic lesion of the right occipital condyle; (b) axial skull base. CT scan with bone window setting showing erosion of the right occipital condyle; (c) right hypoglossal paralysis. Reproduced with permission from Moris G, Roig C, Misiego M, *et al*. The distinctive headache of the occipital condyle syndrome: A report of four cases. *Headache* 1998;38:308–11

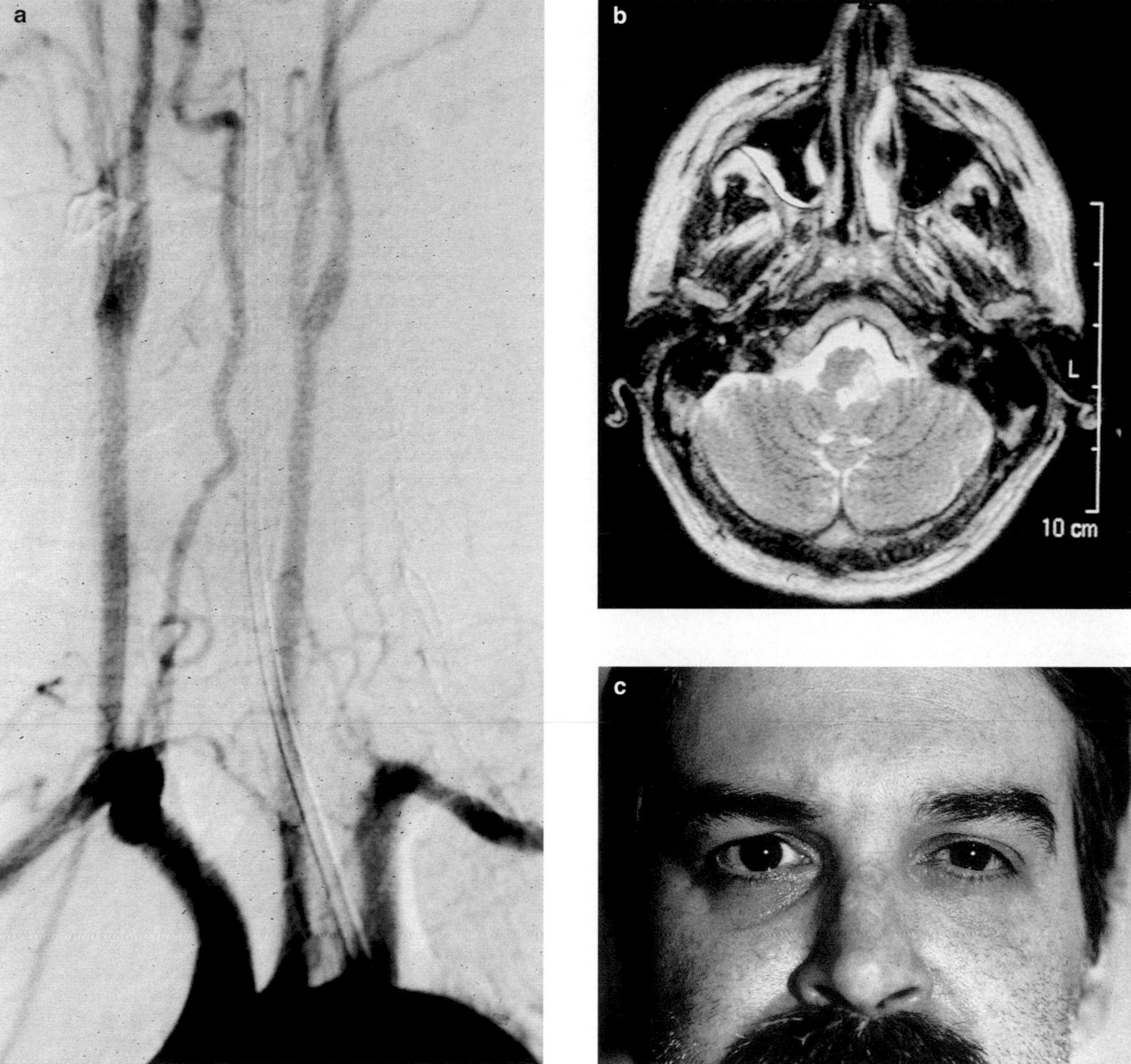


**Figure 8.31** (a), (b) and (c) are from the same patient, a 37-year-old with Wallenberg's syndrome accompanied by retro-ocular headache with autonomic features resembling 'continuous' cluster headache. This case suggests that all the symptomatology typical of cluster headache can be secondary to a pure central lesion. (a) Angiography showing an occlusion of the left vertebral artery, with no sign of dissection; (b) T2-weighted MRI showing an infarct of the left posterior inferior cerebellar artery (PICA) territory; (c) close-up picture of the patient's face showing left palpebral ptosis and conjunctival injection. Reproduced from Cid C, Berciano J, Pascual J. Retro-ocular headache with autonomic features resembling 'continuous' cluster headache in lateral medullary infarction. *J Neurol Neurosurg Psychiatr* 2000;69:134–41, with permission by the BMJ Publishing Group

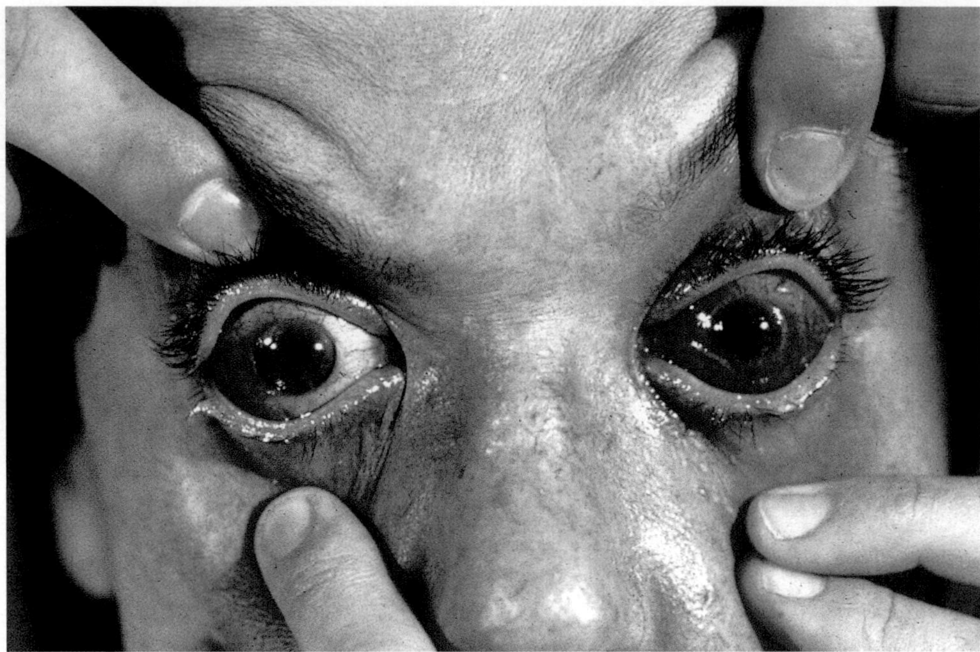

**Figure 8.32** Very severe conjunctival injection (more pronounced in the patient's left side) and uveitis in a 63-year-old woman presenting as bilateral periocular headache as the first sign of a confirmed Wegener's syndrome. Headache and ocular manifestations resolved after aggressive treatment with steroids and cyclophosphamide. Reproduced with kind permission of Julio Pascual

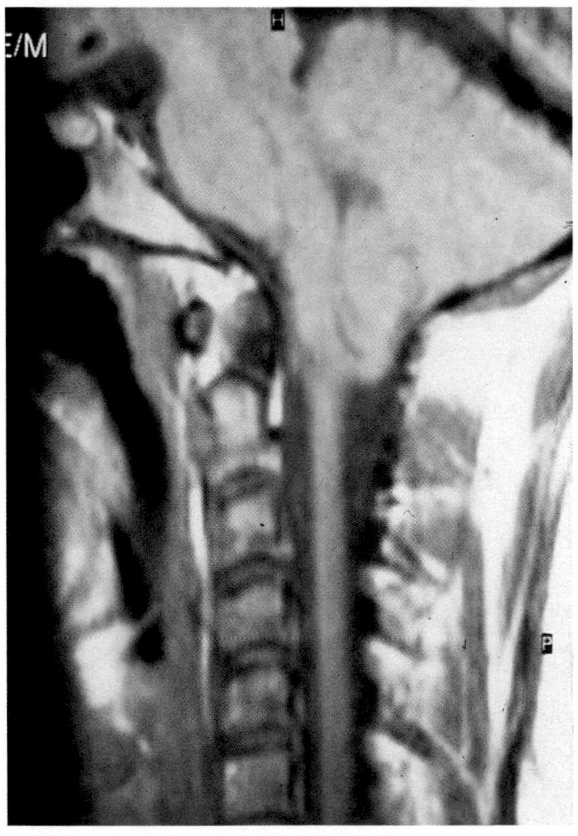

**Figure 8.33** Cranio-cervical MRI study showing tonsillar descent in a 39-year-old woman complaining of brief (second–1 minute) occipital headache when coughing and other Valsalva maneuvers. Sagittal MRI T1 W1 pulse sequence demonstrates low lying tonsils, normal fourth ventricle and normal posterior fossae anatomy indicative of Chiari I. Headache has disappeared after suboccipital craniectomy. Reproduced with permission from Pascual J, Iglesias F, Oterino A, *et al*. Cough, exertional and sexual headache. *Neurology* 1996;46:1520–4

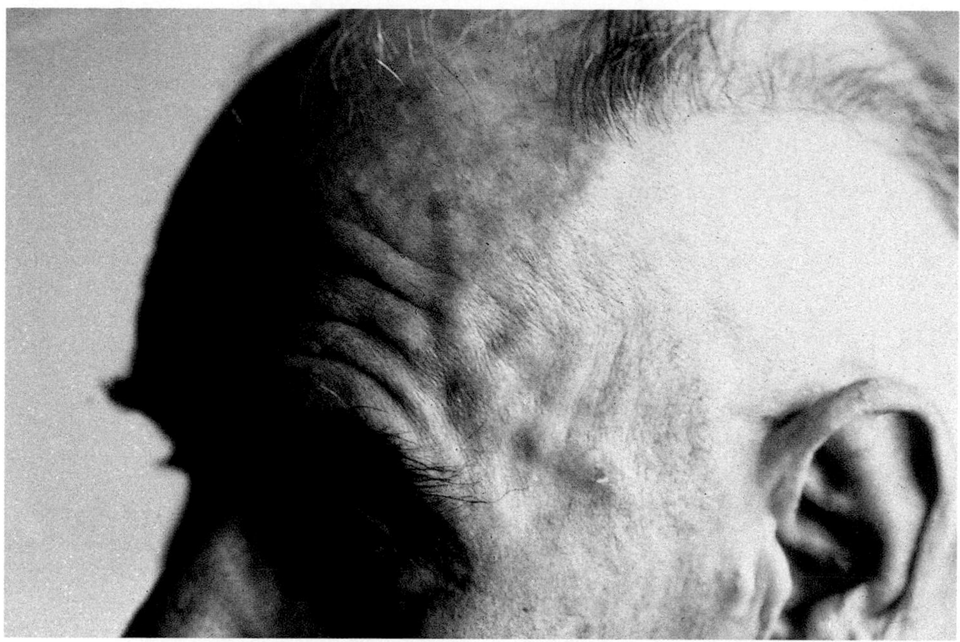

**Figure 8.34** This 78-year-old man went to hospital due to constant temporal headache during the previous two months. On examination there was no pulsation in the left temporal artery, which appeared thickened and painful on palpation. The erythrocyte sedimentation rate was 96 mm in the first hour, while a temporal artery biopsy showed changes diagnostic of giant-cell arteritis. Courtesy of José Berciano, University Hospital Marques de Valdecilla, Santander, Spain

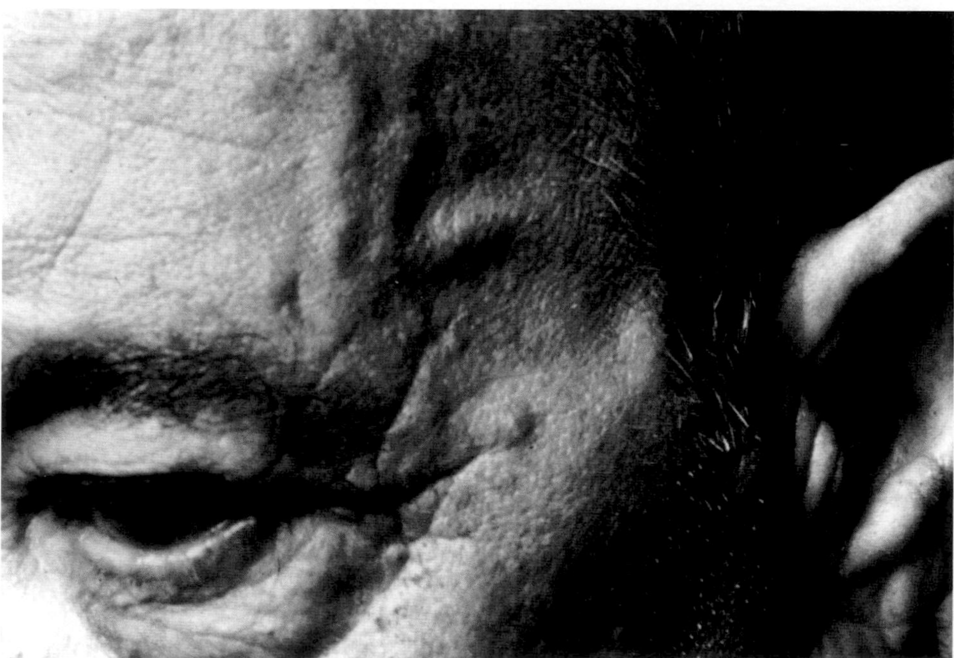

**Figure 8.35** Seventy-year-old man with giant-cell arteritis. A portion of the anterior branch of the left temporal artery is visibly swollen. It was tender and thickened on palpation. Reproduced with permission from Caselli RJ, Hunder GG. Giant cell arteritis and polymyalgia rheumatica. In: Silberstein SD, Lipton RB, Dalessio DJ, eds. *Wolff's Headache and other Head Pain*, 7th edn. New York: Oxford University Press, 2001:525–35

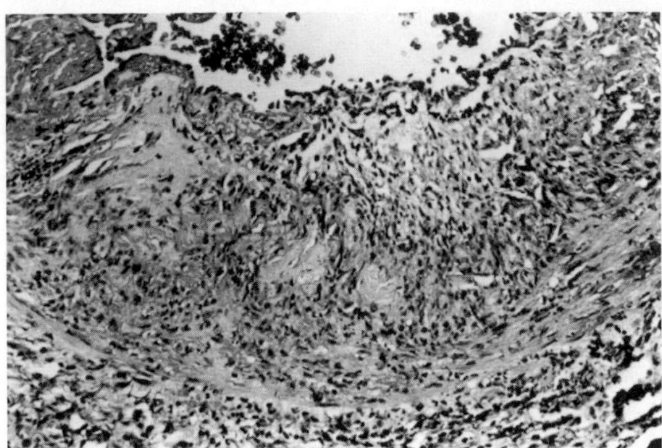

**Figure 8.36** Temporal artery biopsy specimen showing active inflammation in all three vascular layers (intima, media, adventitia). The lumen is partially shown, at the top of the figure, and is narrowed. In most temporal artery biopsy specimens with giant-cell arteritis, the media, especially the inner media in the region of the internal elastic lamina, is involved to the greatest extent and the intimal and adventitial layers are involved to a lesser degree than in this patient (hematoxylin and eosin stain, 200x). Reproduced with permission from Casselli RJ, Hunder GG. Giant cell arteritis and polymyalgia rheumatica. In: Silberstein SD. Lipton RB, Dalessio DJ, eds. *Wolff's Headache and Other Head Pain*, 7th edn. New York: Oxford University Press, 2001:525–35

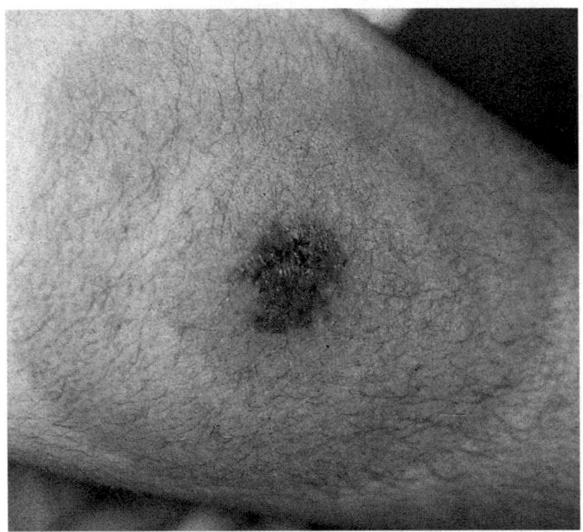

**Figure 8.37** Lyme disease most often presents with a characteristic 'bull's eye' rash, erythema migrans, accompanied by non-specific symptoms such as fever, malaise, fatigue, myalgia and joint aches (arthralgia). Many patients complain of persistent daily headaches

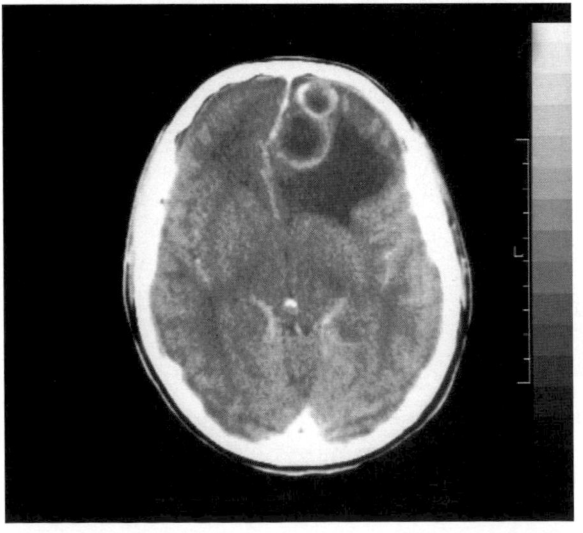

**Figure 8.38** A 22-year-old man with a 1-month history of left hemicranial pain and cluster-like features. An axial CT scan post-enhancement demonstrated a multilocular lesion in the left frontal lobe with white matter edema, displacement of the falx to the right and enhancement of the rings measuring 3.5 cm at the widest. This is a pyogenic brain abscess approximately 14 days old. Reproduced with kind permission of Germany Goncalves Veloso

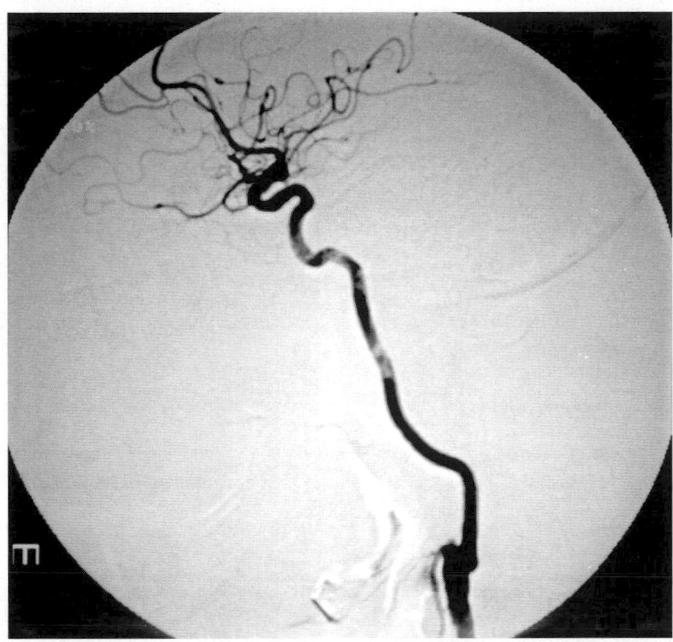

**Figure 8.39** A 53-year-old female patient with a strong pain in the left periocular and temporal region. She presented with autonomic signs, eyelid ptosis and conjunctival injection, ipsilateral to and concurrent with the pain. The duration of the pain was 40 min. It occurred three times per day and was worse at night. As a result of the painful episodes she had decreased sensitivity in the left facial region. The angiogram disclosed an occlusion at the proximal region of the external carotid artery on the left. Patient experienced total relief using verapamil. Reproduced with kind permission of Vera Lucia Faria Xavier

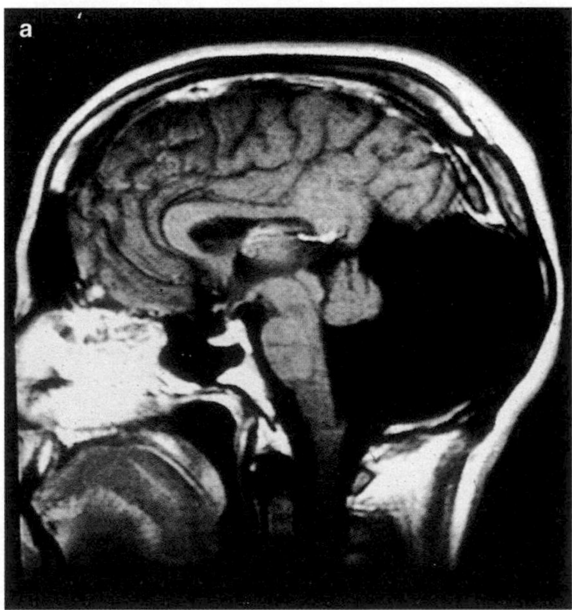

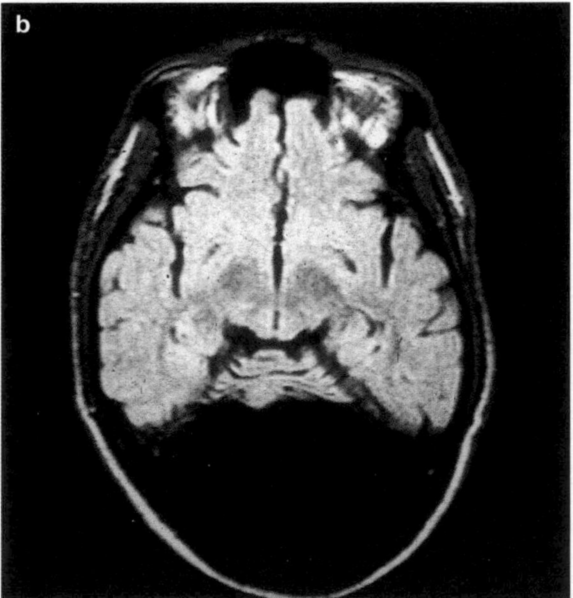

**Figure 8.40** A 34-year-old healthy farmer reported a mild occipital headache for 4 weeks. The general and neurologic examinations were normal. (a) Sagittal T1 W1 MRI and (b) axial T1 W1 MRI showed a large cyst in the posterior fossa displacing the cerebellar hemispheres upwards; this is likely to be a congenital Dandy–Walker abnormality. Surgical approaches were contraindicated by the neurosurgical staff. After 3 years the patient remains asymptomatic, except for transient, mild headaches associated with emotional stress. Reproduced with kind permission of Pericles de Andrade Maranhão-Filho

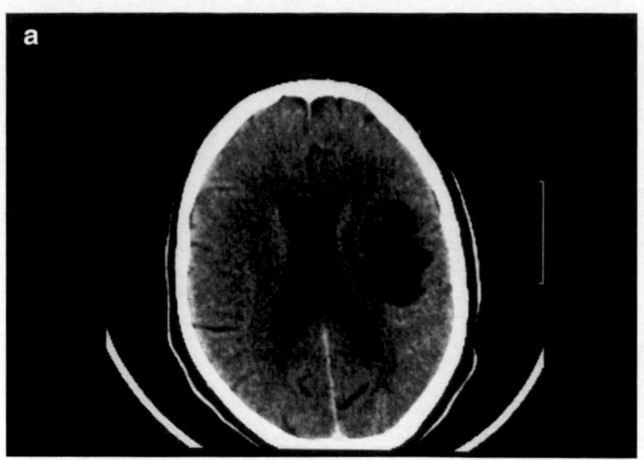

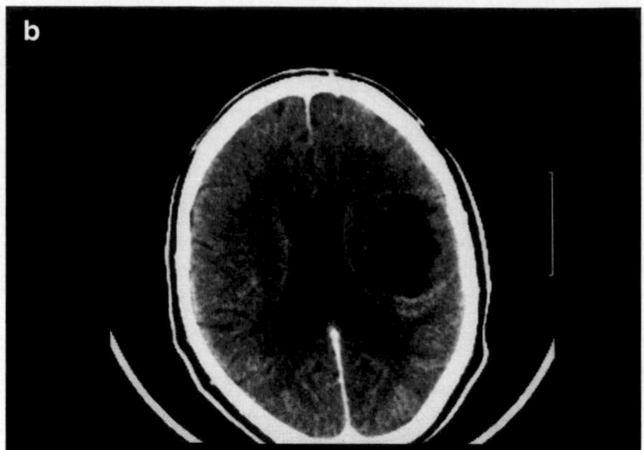

**Figure 8.41** A 35-year-old man with a history of chronic daily headache and recent-onset partial motor seizures. (a) Axial CT scan shows multiloculated cysts in the left sylvian fissure; (b) axial CT scan at the same level. The subarachnoid lesion is not enhanced. The diagnosis is cysticercosis. Reproduced with kind permission of Suzana M F Malheiros

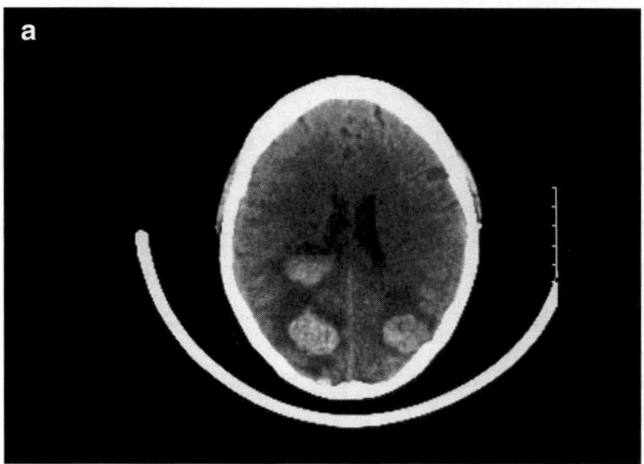

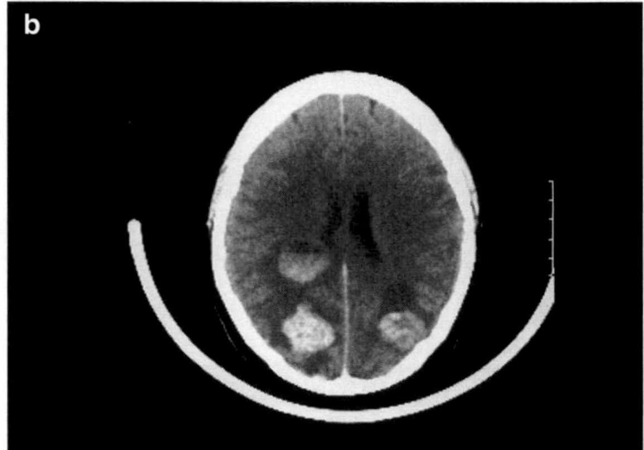

**Figure 8.42** A 34-year-old woman with a history of thunderclap headache during sport activity associated with blurred vision. (a) Axial CT scan shows multifocal high-density intraparenchymal lesions; (b) CT scan shows an irregularly enhancing rim of the three lesions each located bilaterally in the parietal lobes with surrounding edema. Note a fluid–fluid level within the right periventricular lesion. The lesions were confirmed as metastatic melanoma. Reproduced with kind permission of Suzana M F Malheiros

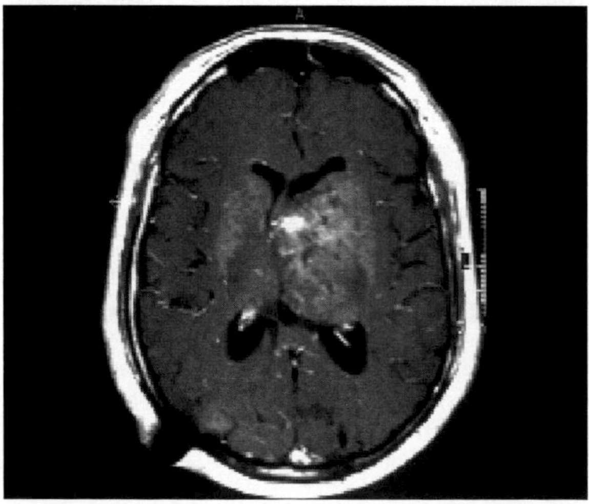

**Figure 8.43** A 60-year-old man with a six-month history of pressing/tightening headache that antedated the development of mild right hemiparesis. Axial post-contrast T1-weighted MR scan shows a large, enhancing, ill-delineated left basal ganglia mass. The diagnosis is anaplastic astrocytoma. Reproduced with kind permission of Suzana M F Malheiros

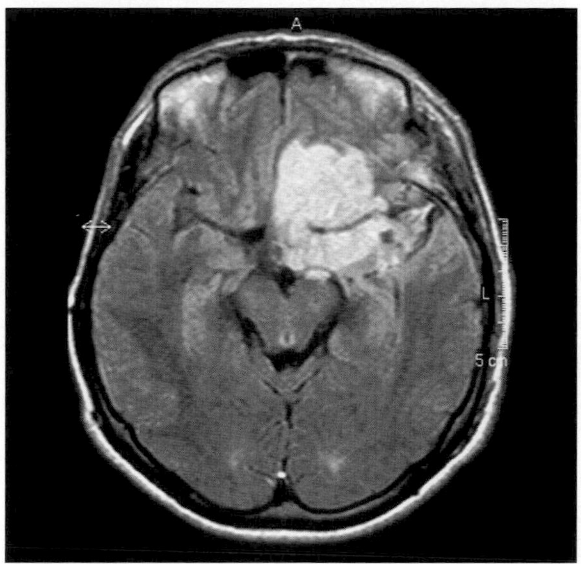


**Figure 8.44** A 29-year-old man with a history of sudden-onset headache associated with exertional worsening. Axial FLAIR image demonstrates a hyperintense left fronto-temporal scallop-bordered mass (approximately 5 × 3.7 cm) well circumscribed with no edema. The diagnosis is primitive neuroendodermal tumor (PNET). Reproduced with kind permission of Suzana M F Malheiros

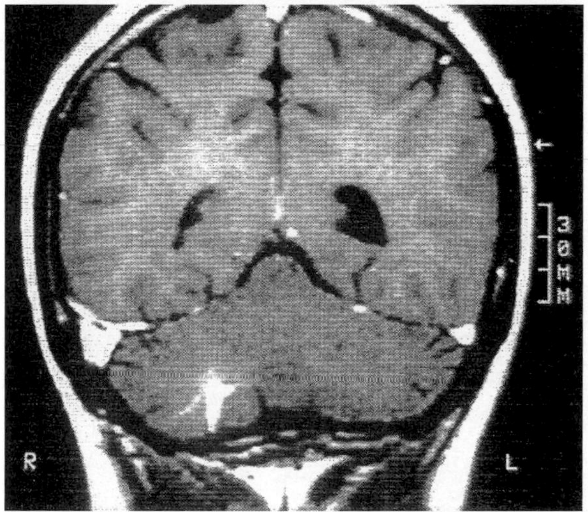


**Figure 8.45** Sagittal T1 W1 MRI post-enhancement venous angioma. A right cerebellar linear enhancing structure with a trans-cerebellar course demonstrating uniform enhancement and classic umbrella shape

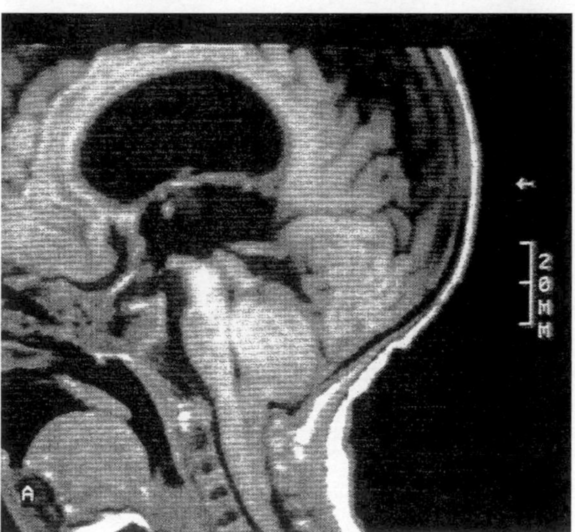


**Figure 8.46** Sagittal T1 W1 non-enhanced MRI demonstrating a Chiari II malformation. Note the low-lying tonsils, flattening of the aqueduct, compression of the fourth ventricle and a widened cervical cord

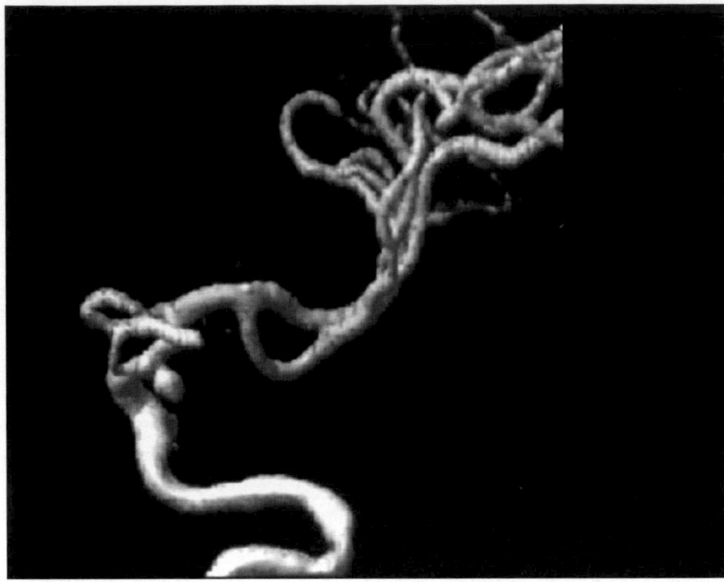

**Figure 8.47** Carotid arteriogram showing an aneurysm which comes to a point consistent with this being the area of pathology. No areas of spasm are noted. Reproduced with kind permission of Nitamar Abdala

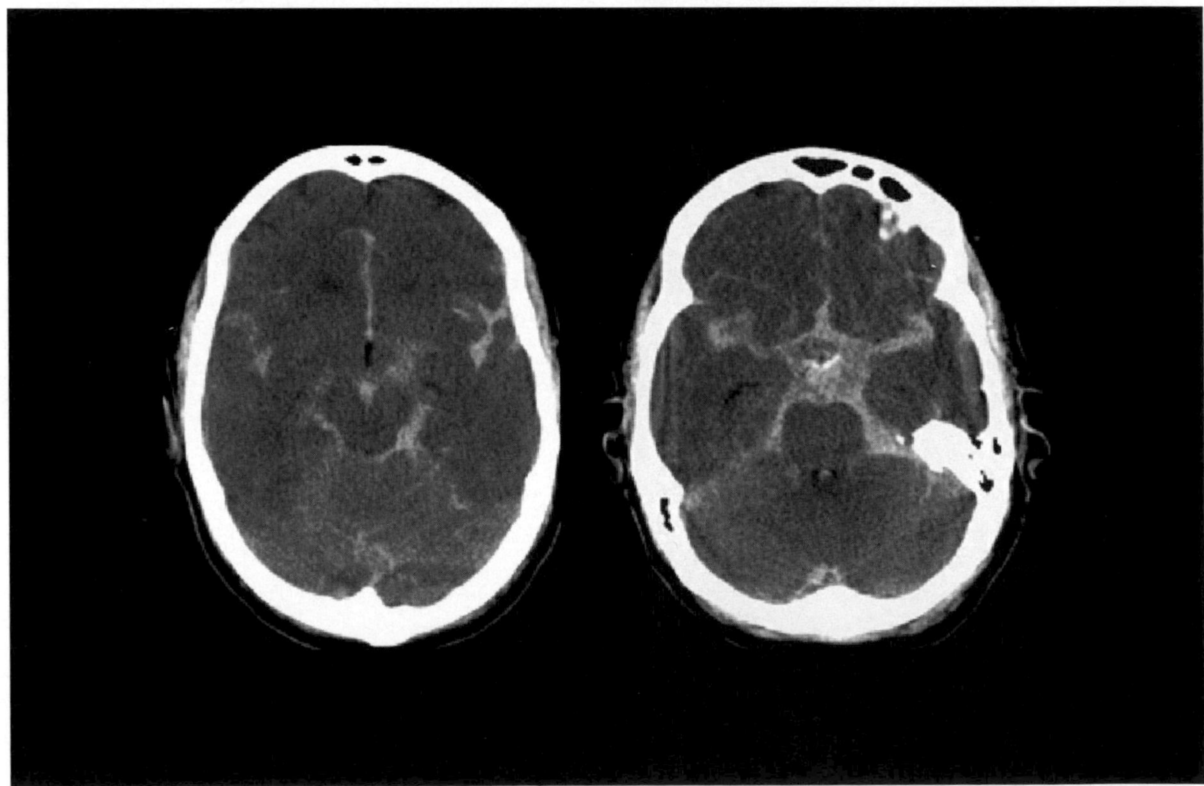

**Figure 8.48** Two axial CT scans showing diffuse blood-filled CSF and cisternal spaces. There is increased density consistent with a diffuse subarachnoid hemorrhage. Reproduced with kind permission of Nitamar Abdala

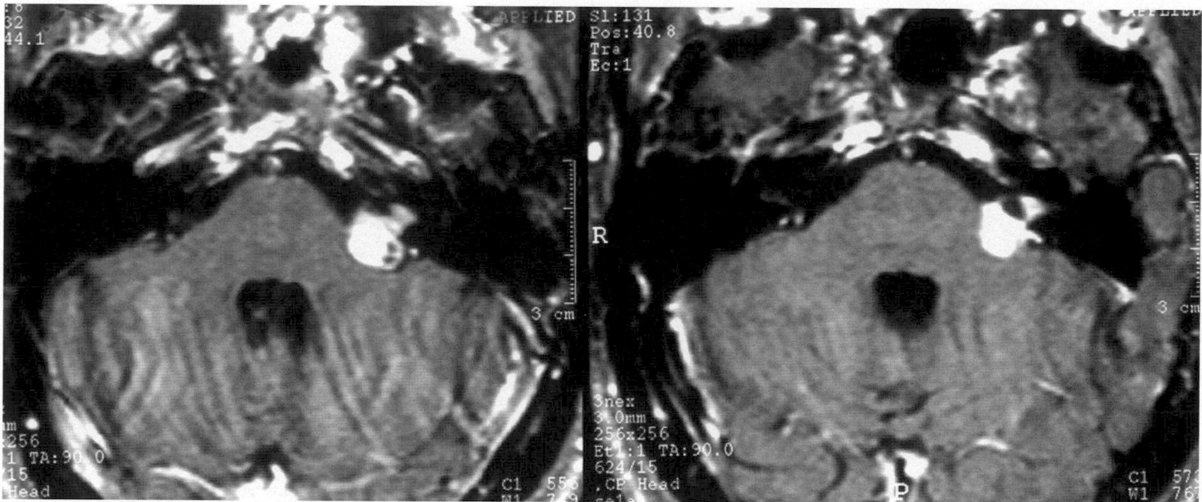


**Figure 8.49** A middle-aged male with left-sided head pain and hearing loss. Two posterior fossae T1 MRI post-enhancement images show a cerebellopontine angle component of 1 cm with an intracanalicular extension. Uniformly enhancing mass with a cisternal and intracanalicular component; widening of the internal auditory canal is consistent with a vestibular schwannoma. Reproduced with kind permission of Nitamar Abdala

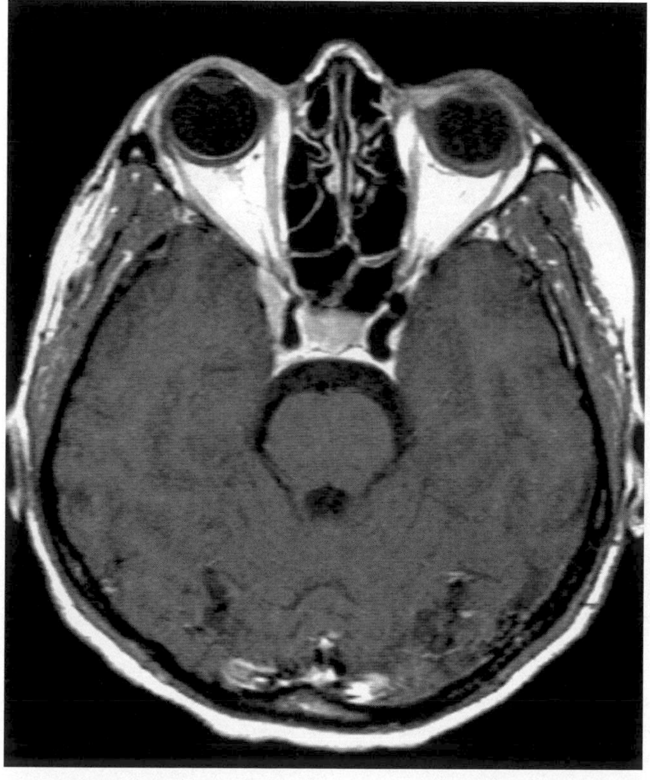

**Figure 8.50** Tolosa-Hunt syndrome is an idiopathic inflammatory condition that usually presents with painful ophthalmoplegia. An axial T1 MRI shows a soft tissue mass filling the lateral aspect of the right cavernous sinus compressing and medially displacing the carotid artery and extruding to the apex of the right orbit. Reproduced with kind permission of Nitamar Abdala

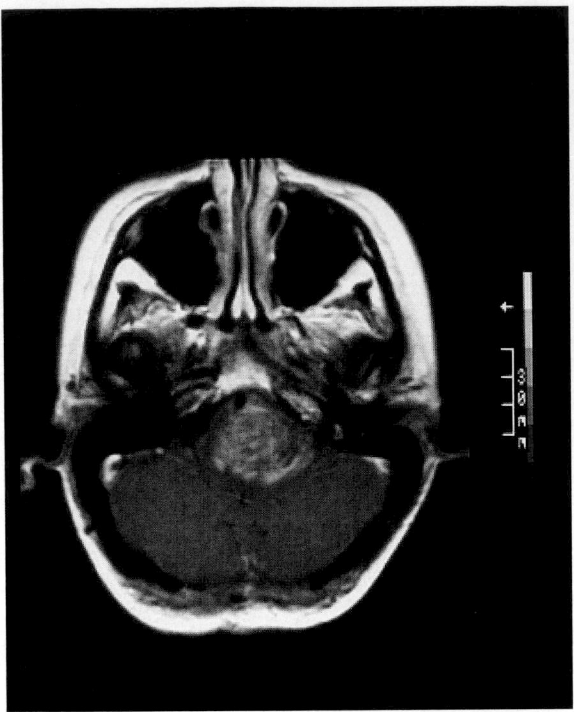

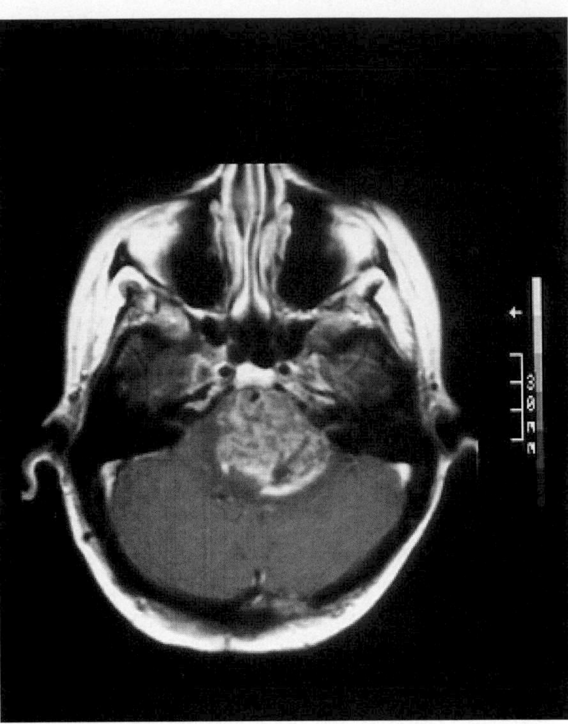

**Figure 8.51** A 32-year-old woman with a four-month history of a new-onset throbbing headache followed by sixth nerve palsy and ataxia. Axial post-contrast T1-weighted MR scans show a large, enhancing, well-delineated mass that expands and distorts the pons. The diagnosis is anaplastic astrocytoma. Reproduced with kind permission of Suzana M F Malheiros

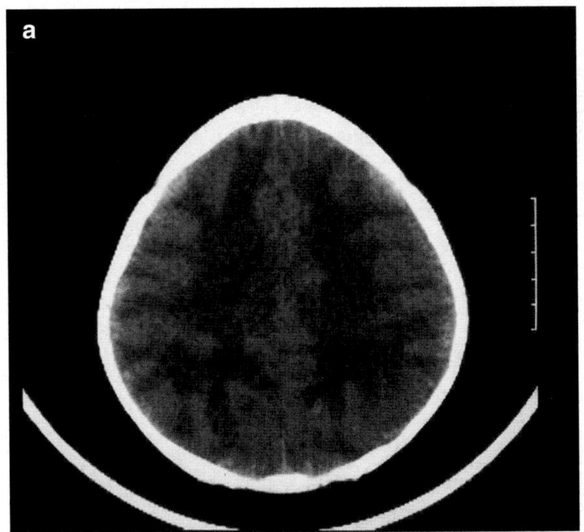


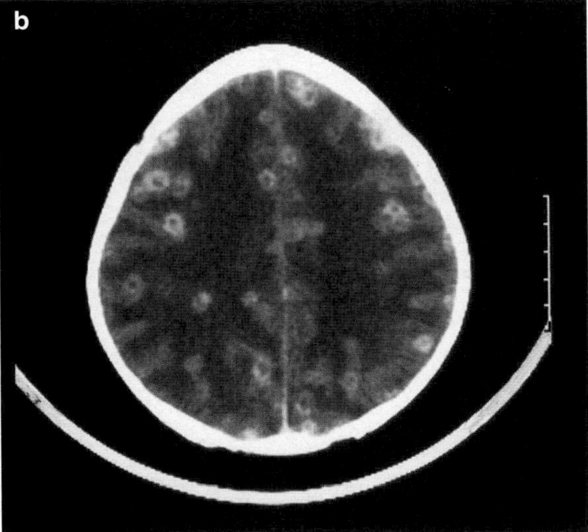


**Figure 8.52** A 15-year-old girl with a history of progressive severe headache initiating 2 weeks before, associated with nausea, vomiting and decreased consciousness. (a) Axial CT scan shows ill-defined low-density changes in the white matter of both hemispheres; (b) axial CT scan at the same level shows multifocal subcortical white matter ring-enhancing lesions. The diagnosis is cysticercosis. Reproduced with kind permission of Suzana M F Malheiros

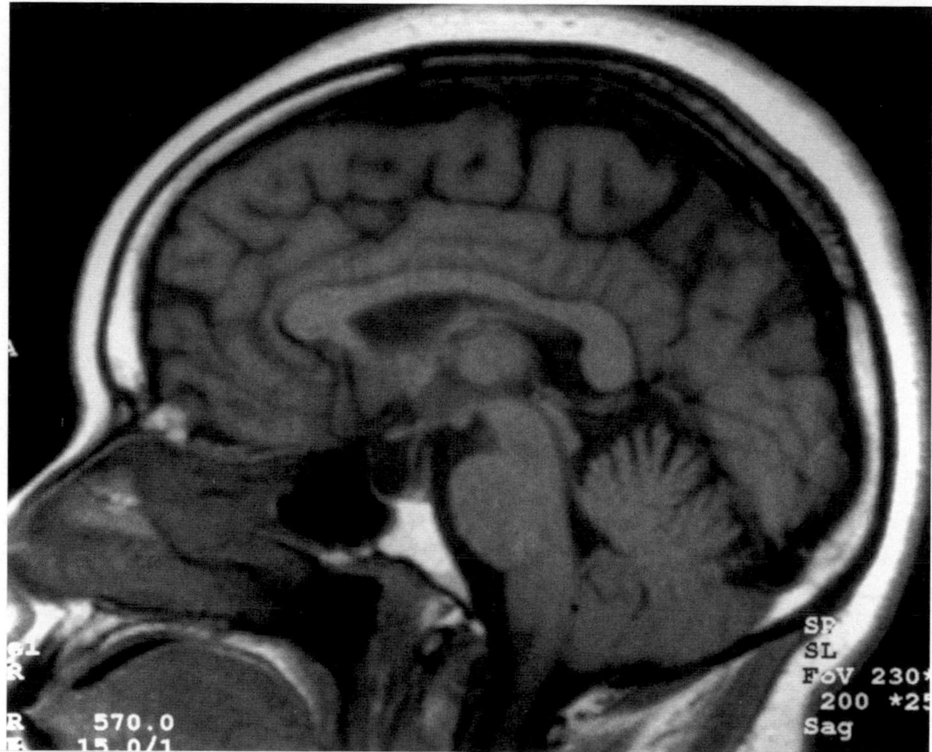


**Figure 8.53** A middle-aged woman presenting with headaches is found to have an empty sella. A sagittal T1 MRI demonstrating a stretched pituitary infundibulum with no significant visible pituitary tissue

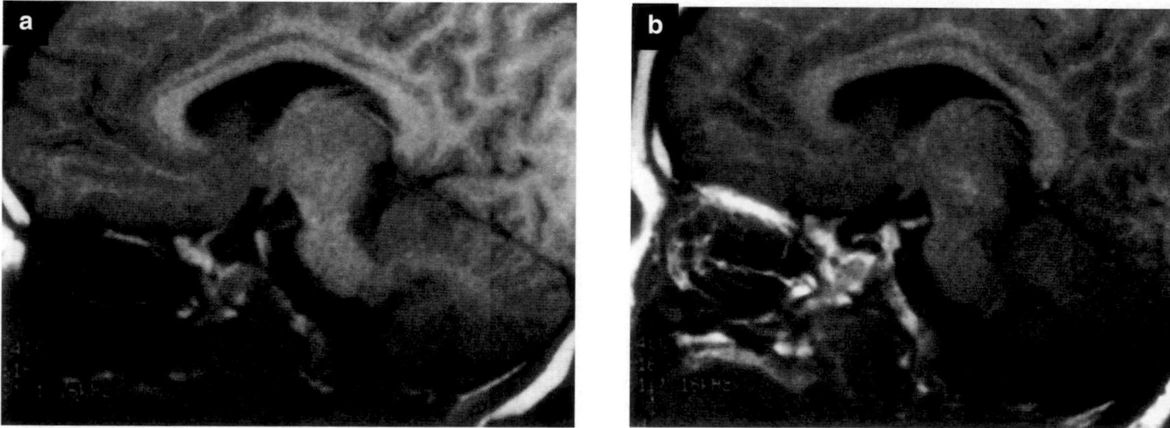


**Figure 8.54** Three-year-old boy with two prior episodes of spontaneously resolving oculomotor nerve palsy. (a) and (b), sagittal T1-weighted MR images before (a) and after (b) contrast administration show diffuse thickening and enhancement of the oculomotor nerve. The symptoms resolved spontaneously in 6 weeks. Reproduced with permission from Mark AS, Casselman J, Brown D, *et al.* Ophthalmoplegic migraine: Reversible enhancement and thickening of the cisternal segment of the oculomotor nerve on contrast-enhanced MR images. *Am J Neuroradiol* 1998;19:1887–91, copyright © American Society of Neuroradiology (www.ajnr.org)

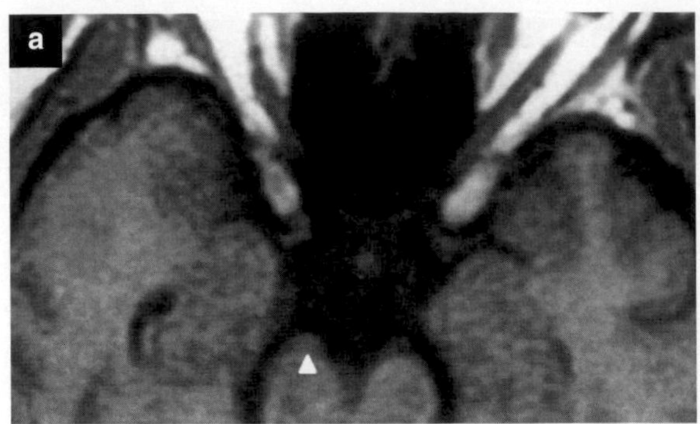

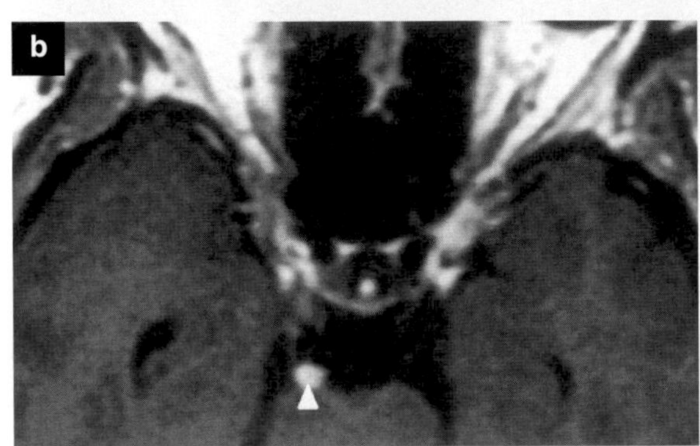

**Figure 8.55** Twenty-seven-year old woman with two prior episodes of headache and oculomotor nerve palsy. (a) and (b), axial non-contrast (a) and contrast-enhanced (b) T1-weighted images show focal nodular enhancement of the exit zone of the oculomotor nerve (see arrows). Follow-up study showed virtually complete resolution of the enhancement. Reproduced with permission from Mark AS, Casselman J, Brown D, *et al.* Ophthalmoplegic migraine: Reversible enhancement and thickening of the cisternal segment of the oculomotor nerve on contrast-enhanced MR images. *Am J Neuroradiol* 1998;19: 1887–91, copyright © American Society of Neuroradiology (www.ajnr.org)

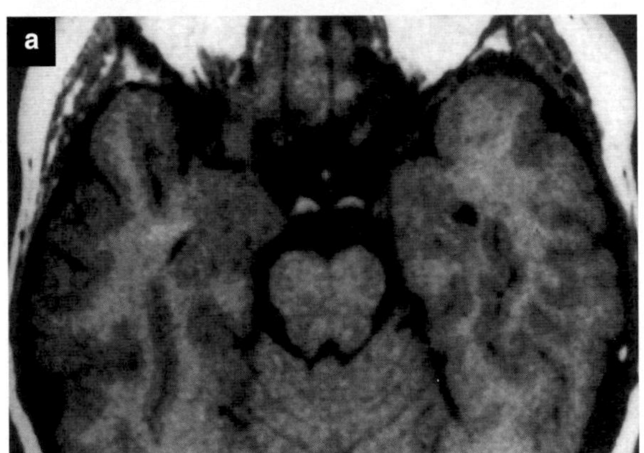

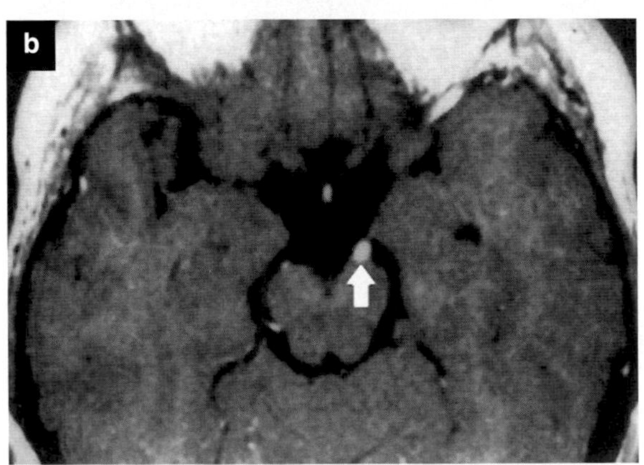

**Figure 8.56** Twelve-year-old boy with two prior episodes of ophthalmoplegic migraine. (a) and (b), axial T1-weighted MR images before (a) and after (b) contrast administration show enhancement of the oculomotor nerve (arrow in panel b) and thickening of its root entry zone. Follow-up studies showed virtually complete resolution of the enhancement. Reproduced with permission from Mark AS, Casselman J, Brown D, *et al.* Ophthalmoplegic migraine: Reversible enhancement and thickening of the cisternal segment of the oculomotor nerve on contrast-enhanced MR images. *Am J Neuroradiol* 1998;19: 1887–91, copyright © American Society of Neuroradiology (www.ajnr.org)

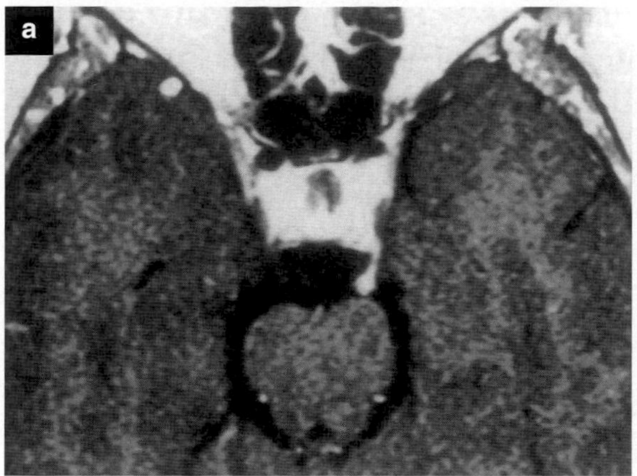

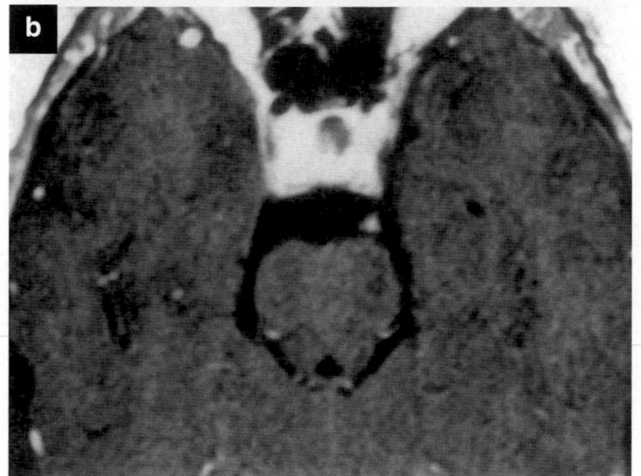

**Figure 8.57** Twenty-three-year-old woman with one prior episode of ophthalmoplegic migraine. (a) axial T1-weighted contrast-enhanced MR image shows enhancement of the oculomotor nerve and thickening of its root entry zone; (b) follow-up study shows virtually complete resolution of the enhancement. Reproduced with permission from Mark AS, Casselman J, Brown D, *et al*. Ophthalmoplegic migraine: Reversible enhancement and thickening of the cisternal segment of the oculomotor nerve on contrast-enhanced MR images. *Am J Neuroradiol* 1998;19:1887–91, copyright © American Society of Neuroradiology (www.ajnr.org)

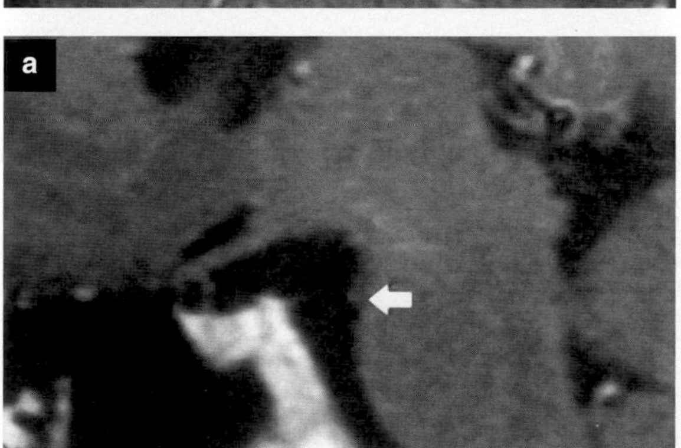

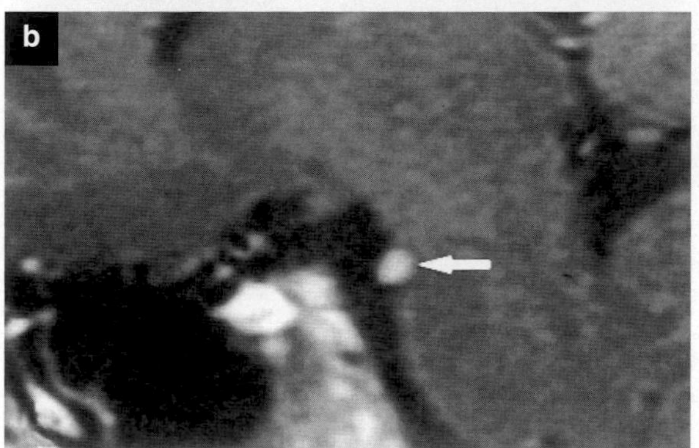

**Figure 8.58** Eight-year-old girl with one prior episode of spontaneously resolving oculomotor nerve palsy. (a) and (b), sagittal T1-weighted MR image before (a) and after (b) contrast administration show focal thickening and enhancement of the root exit zone (see arrows). The symptoms resolved spontaneously within 6 weeks. Reproduced with permission from Mark AS, Casselman J, Brown D, *et al*. Ophthalmoplegic migraine: Reversible enhancement and thickening of the cisternal segment of the oculomotor nerve on contrast-enhanced MR images. *Am J Neuroradiol* 1998;19:1887–91, copyright © American Society of Neuroradiology (www.ajnr.org)

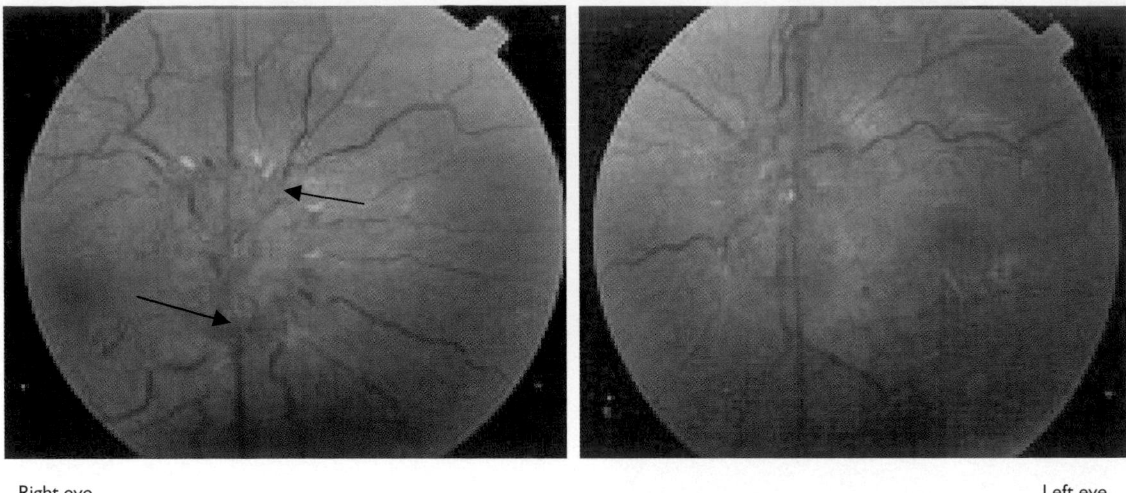


**Figure 8.59** Marked papilledema (Frisén Stage 4[7]). Features that determine the severity of papilledema are optic disc elevation, obliteration of optic cup, a peripapillary halo, and disappearance of one or more vessels crossing the optic disc margin (arrows). Vascular tortuosity is generally present. This patient also has nerve fiber layer hemorrhages and exudates, arranged radially around the disc border in the right eye. Courtesy of D Friedman

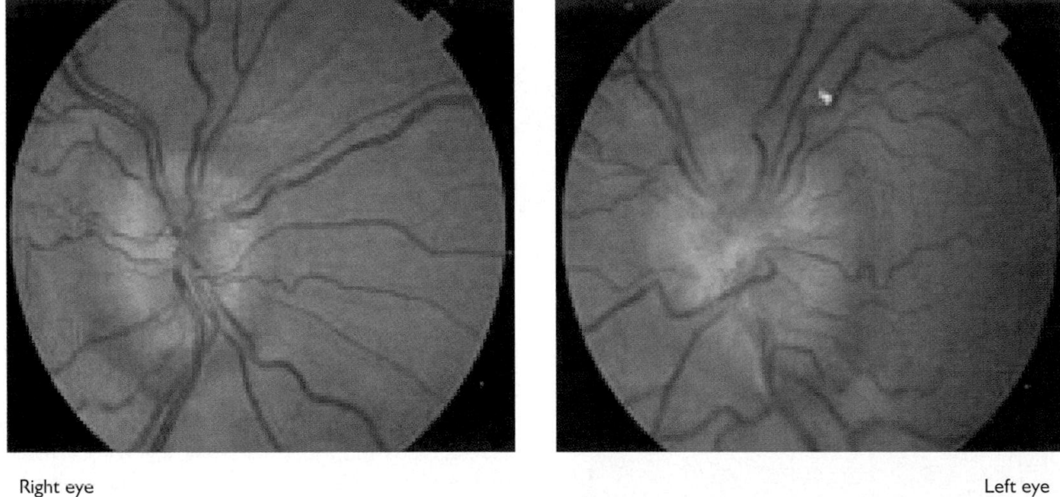


**Figure 8.60** Pseudotumor cerebri. A 16-year-old with lymphoma and superior sagittal sinus thrombosis developed papilledema without visual loss. Note the diffuse disc elevation and peripapillary halo surrounding the optic nerve. All vessels are seen crossing the disc margin (early papilledema, Frisén Stage 2[7]). The papilledema resolved with diuretic treatment and the lymphoma was successfully treated. Courtesy of D Friedman

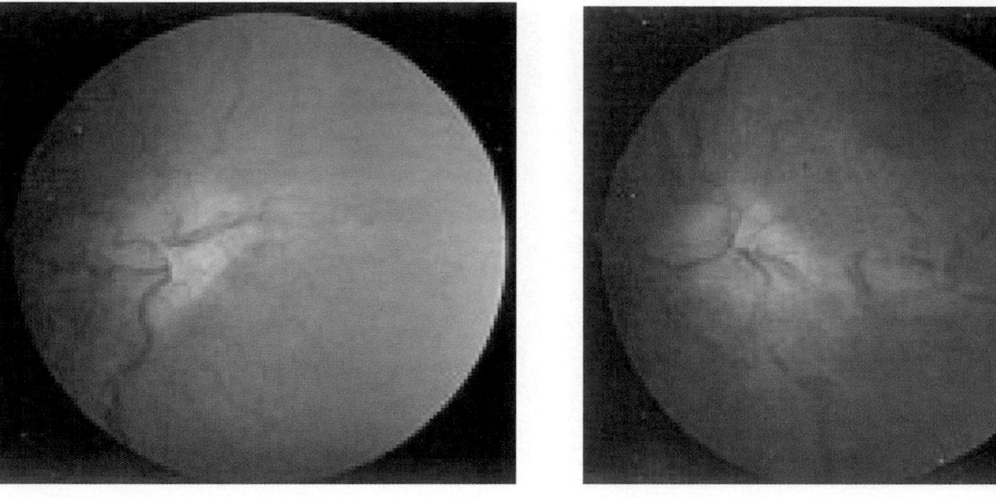


**Figure 8.61** A 40-year-old woman was hospitalized for $CO_2$ retention and cor pulmonale. There was a 10-year history of gradual weight gain (weight >350 lb). She had progressive visual loss with papilledema while in the hospital, not responsive to bilateral optic nerve sheath fenestration which was performed under local anesthesia because of her respiratory problems. Portable fundus photography showed pale, swollen optic nerves with obscuration of vessels crossing the disc margins and obliteration of the optic cup (severe papilledema, Frisén Stage 5[7]). The patient refused intubation and died. Courtesy of D Friedman

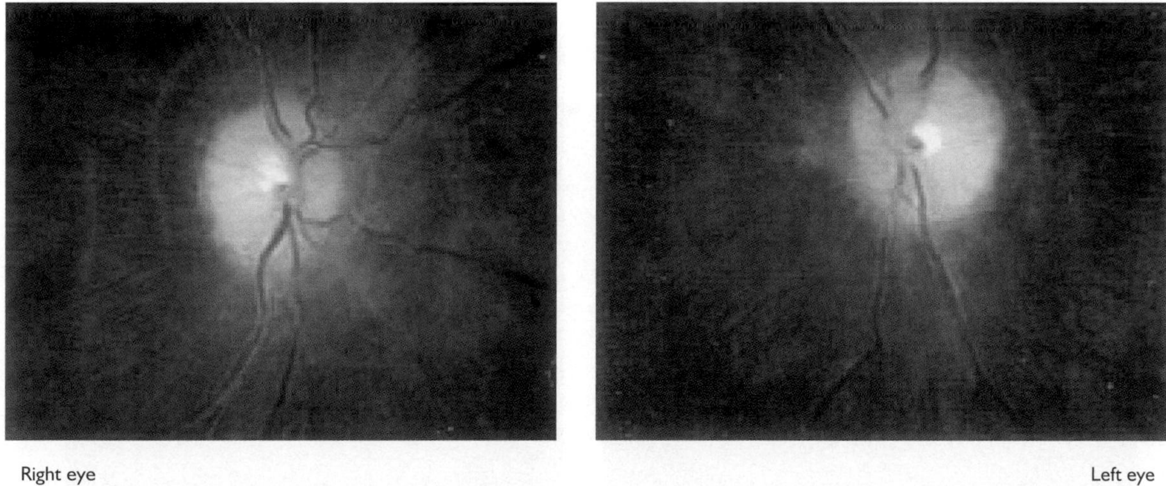


**Figure 8.62** A short 5-year-old girl had headaches, bilateral papilledema, and 20/80 vision in both eyes. Idiopathic intracranial hypertension was diagnosed and she was treated with acetazolamide. She did not return for follow-up until several months later when her acuity had declined to 20/200 OU. A lumboperitoneal shunt was inserted without substantial improvement in her vision. Endocrinologic evaluation revealed Turner syndrome. Her optic nerves are pale and atrophic with gliosis of the peripapillary nerve fiber layer. Courtesy of D Friedman

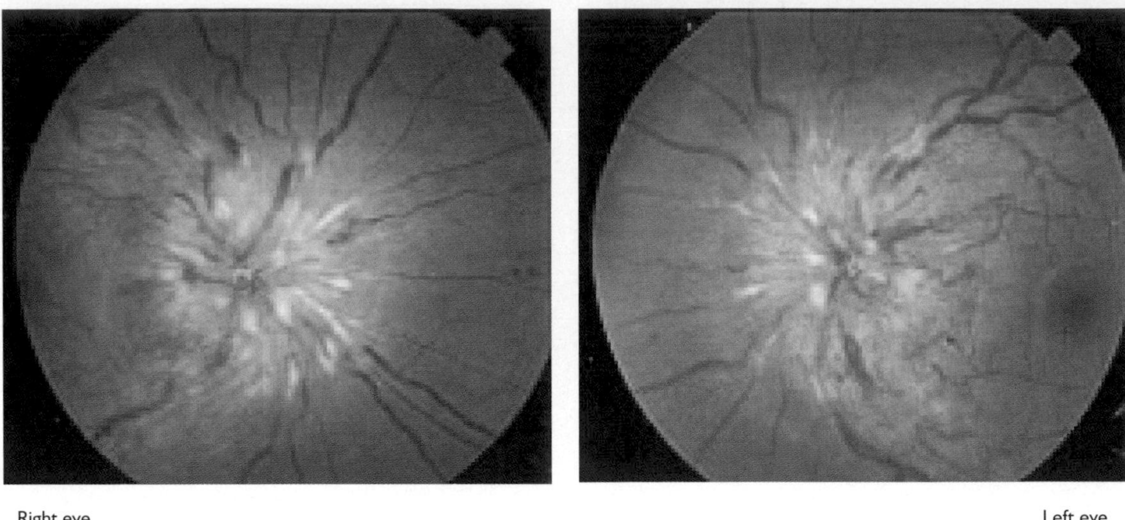


**Figure 8.63** A 19-year-old woman had a six-week history of worsening headaches, diplopia and visual loss. Examination revealed bilateral VI nerve palsies, marked visual field constriction (OS>OD) and papilledema. There is severe papilledema with anterior expansion of the optic nerve head, loss of the optic cup and disappearance of major blood vessels crossing the disc. She has pronounced nerve fiber layer hemorrhages and exudates. She was treated with optic nerve sheath fenestration OS and acetazolamide, with improvement in her vision and papilledema, but sustained permanent visual field loss. Courtesy of D Friedman

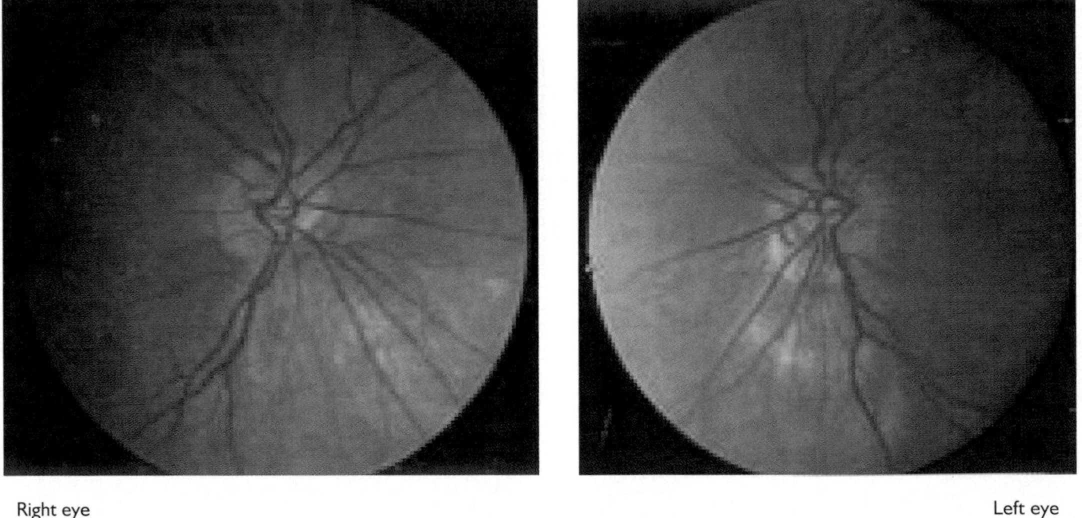


**Figure 8.64** Tilted optic discs (pseudopapilledema). Tilted optic discs are a congenital variation that may be present in nearsighted individuals. Unlike true papilledema, the temporal margin of the disc often appears more swollen than the nasal margin. Their presence in a patient with chronic headaches may simulate pseudotumor cerebri. Courtesy of D Friedman

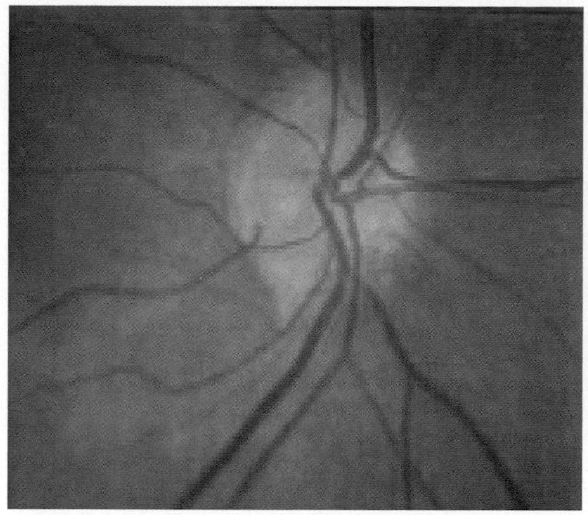

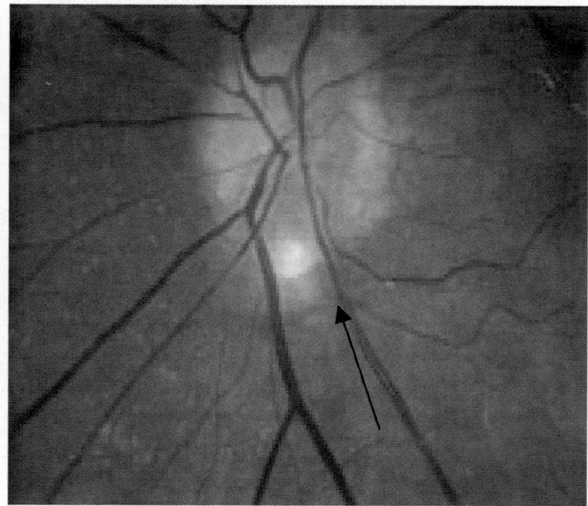

Right eye    Left eye

**Figure 8.65** Optic disc drusen (pseudopapilledema). Optic disc drusen are calcifications that lie on or below the surface of the optic nerve. They cause a 'lumpy-bumpy' appearance of the nerve that may be difficult to distinguish from disc swelling on direct ophthalmoscopy. Sometimes the calcifications are obvious (arrow) but ultrasound or computed tomography may be needed to diagnose deeper ('buried') drusen. Courtesy of D Friedman

ered a strong diagnostic indicator of a primary headache because organic disease may cause migrainous symptoms. Most problematic are the patients with neurologic disorders who present with headache in isolation, not necessarily accompanied by neurologic abnormalities on examination. The age of onset, precipitating or aggravating factors, and change in headache pattern may assist the clinician in deciding the need for neurodiagnostic testing. However the final outcome will undoubtedly depend on the physician's knowledge of the IHS classification, a comfort level with the so-called red flags, and close monitoring of the patient's symptoms and signs upon presentation and after treatment. Unfortunately, the causes of secondary headaches are too numerous to discuss in detail. The images included with the text (Figures 8.1–8.65) help to elucidate just how varied the secondary causes can be.

## REFERENCES


1. Headache Classification Subcommittee of the International Headache Society. The International Classification of Headache Disorders, 2nd edn. *Cephalalgia* 2004;24(Suppl 1):1–150
2. Edmeads J. Challenges in the diagnosis of acute headache. Headache 1999;2:537–40
3. Lewis BW. Qureschis. Acute headache in children and adolescents presenting to ED. *Headache* 2000; 40:25–9
4. Medina LS, *et al.* Children with headache: clinical predictors of surgical space occupying lesions and the role of neuroimaging. *Radiology* 1997;202: 819–24
5. Silberstein, S D. An evidence based review: practice parameters evidence based guidelines for migraine headache. US Headache Consortium. *Neurology* 2000;55:754–63
6. Quality Standard Subcommittee of the American Academy of Neurology. Practice parameter: the utility of neuroimaging in the evaluation of headache in patients with normal neurologic examination. *Neurology* 1994;44:1191–7
7. Frisén L. Swelling of the optic nerve head. A staging scheme. *J Neurol Neurosurg Psychiatry* 1982;45: 13–18

# Index